HEMP HEALTH
REVOLUTION

The A to Z
Health Benefits
of Hemp Extract

Dr. Sherrill Sellman, N.D.

D0976304

HEMP HEALTH REVOLUTION

IMOV LLC
825 East 800 North
Orem, UT 84097

Publisher:
Elite Online Publishing
63 East 11400 South #230
Sandy, UT 84070
www.EliteOnlinePublishing.com

ISBN-13: 978-1981459629
ISBN-10: 1981459626

CONTENTS

PREFACE

As a medical practitioner dedicated to seeking the most effective solutions to the many health challenges that are facing our modern world, I have realized that the truth is often both apparent and hidden from us.

A major way that pharmaceutical companies find new drugs is by examining chemicals provided by nature that have existed for millennia in plants, but then altering those already effective chemicals, not necessarily to make them better, but to be able to patent them.

The world of hemp research to scientifically validate the effectiveness of natural cannabinoid molecular extracts to promote various aspects of health that has been known to ancient cultures for millennia is a prime example of this. Pharmaceutical companies are actively researching these same and very effective natural chemicals to be able to patent altered versions under obscure trade names. However, the pure, natural, and safe extracts of this amazing plant are finally being made available to us and again being recognized for their powerful healing qualities.

For decades, the healing gifts of this plant were maligned and demonized. Farmers were forbidden from growing hemp. Even more sinister, anyone who needed the medicinal benefits was labeled a criminal and risked incarceration. This banishment of the amazing hemp plant had much more to do with ignorance, politics and corporate interests than the health and welfare of society.

I am truly excited to see that we are finally regaining the knowledge and appreciation of just how profound this plant can be for our health. Hemp extract has been shown to help alleviate chronic pain and reduce epileptic seizures, depression, anxiety, insomnia and stress. Further studies are revealing that hemp extract is beneficial for autoimmune diseases. In addition to its well-known help in reducing adverse side effects of cancer treatments such as nausea, it has shown promise as a cancer treatment in and of itself. The more science investigates hemp extract, the more their discoveries reveal the many gifts that are found hidden within this amazing plant.

Compared to the many serious side effects from pharmaceutical drugs, we can be especially grateful that the veil on the many secrets found within the hemp plant is being lifted, and knowledge such as that being well-presented in this book is being spread.

Ron Rosedale M.D., author of *The Rosedale Diet*
www.DrRosedale.com

Hemp is now in the public consciousness in ways that it has never been before; it seems that news stories and scientific studies are continuously coming out. However, the real question is, what is the benefit, and how can it be used by us to enjoy its myriad of potential benefits? Dr. Sellman puts together a comprehensive yet straightforward and easy-to-understand guide to this subject matter so that we can enjoy the benefits.

As always, Dr. Sellman introduces the cutting edge in this field and includes a section on a natural yet advanced nutrient delivery system using liposomes. HempSorb™, as its name suggests, is designed to get the hemp to absorb rather than just pass through your body. This advanced system wraps around the hemp oil and naturally helps it to be more fully absorbed and then utilized by your body. Remember that no absorption equals no benefits.

Dr. Emek Blair, Ph.D. in Bio-Analytical Chemistry at
The University of California – Irvine (UC)
Award winner for his work on enzymes and lipids. Discoverer of all-natural methods of creating liposomes.

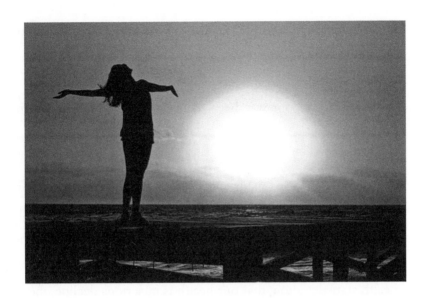

"All that man needs for health and healing has been provided by God in nature; the challenge of science is to find it."

- Paracelsus

CHAPTER 1: WAKING UP TO THE HEALING POWER OF THE HEMP PLANT

We live in a time of profound transformation. More and more people are questioning their reliance on pharmaceutical drugs while also searching for safer and more effective alternatives.

It is obvious that we urgently need new solutions to the health crisis facing our society.

It's time to find our way back to health by reconnecting to nature's healing energies.

Although we are a wealthy nation, we are poverty-stricken when it comes to our health. Compared with other developed and many developing nations, the United States continues to rank at or near the bottom in indicators of mortality and life expectancy. While our health statistics show that our health is in serious decline, the amount paid for healthcare far exceeds other countries in per capita health spending.

We are facing an epidemic of chronic diseases. There are now 133 million Americans – 45% of the population – that have at least one chronic disease.

Seven out of every 10 deaths are due to chronic illnesses. That means 1.7 million people die annually from some type of chronic condition.

Future predictions tell us that by 2025, nearly half of the entire population of the US, 164 million people, will be diagnosed with a chronic disease.

That means that nearly half of the US population will be facing the following chronic illnesses:

Arthritis

Autism

Autoimmune issues

Cancer

Dementia

Depression

Diabetes

Heart disease

Neurodegenerative diseases (Parkinson's or Alzheimer's)

Obesity

Psychiatric conditions

Strokes

Relying on the traditional medical approach is failing us. At best, pharmaceutical interventions may reduce symptoms. But they are always accompanied by a plethora of side effects, which adds to more complications.

Pharmaceutical drugs never really heal the body. They never get to the root cause of the illness, nor do they resolve the underlying imbalance. And chances are their side effects will contribute to even more serious health problems.

The health transformation that is now happening is really a wake-up call. We are arriving at the realization that the solutions we are seeking to our health problems are not found in the labs of major pharmaceutical companies but rather in nature. It's not about manipulation of biochemical processes but rather restoration of homeostasis, the inner balance and harmony within our body that underlies health.

Nature is the source of the healing energy that allows us to truly align with health and optimal wellness. For thousands of years and throughout the world, nature has worked her magic through plants. There is a huge repository of knowledge pertaining to the therapeutic use of medicinal plants.

Through the advancement of science, recent discoveries have unlocked the healing secret of one particular ancient medicinal plant.

The hemp plant, cannabis sativa, has powerful healing, non-psychoactive constituents, known as cannabinoids or Hemp Extract, that are capable of restoring balance and harmony throughout the body without any known side effects. It was discovered that this amazing plant is able to restore the body to inner balance, or homeostasis, through a newly discovered system in the body called the endocannabinoid system.

The purpose of this book is to explain the emerging science of cannabinoids and, in particular, Hemp Extract and its many proven healing benefits.

This is an exciting and expanding area of research as more and more scientists from around the world discover the many chronic diseases and health conditions that can be safely and successfully resolved by using Hemp Extract, orally as well as topically.

The good news is that children as well as adults can benefit from using Hemp Extract.

It's important to emphasize the point that we are talking about the non-psychoactive components of the agricultural hemp plant, not medical marijuana. These are two totally different forms of the cannabis plant with a different biochemical makeup.

You may be wondering about the legality of Hemp Extract, which is derived from agricultural hemp. The good news is that it is totally legal in all 50 states.

The healing benefits from Hemp Extract also extend into the animal world. Our pets can safely benefit from taking it as well. Cats and dogs are mirroring our patterns of chronic illnesses. What's more, veterinary clinics are now supplied with their own pharmacopeia of powerful and potentially toxic medications. Fortunately, our furry friends have a natural option that can help them to get healthy.

This book explores the latest research in Hemp Extract. Most importantly, I will list the many chronic illnesses or health conditions that have been proven to benefit from Hemp Extract.

But you don't need to be sick to benefit from Hemp Extract. It also bestows many anti-aging benefits such as stress reduction, improved sleep, balanced moods, immune support, hormonal balance and much more.

I think you will be amazed, as I have been, to learn about Hemp Extract's many healing secrets. To a world greatly in need of an effective, natural remedy without known side effects, the discovery of Hemp Extract is truly a godsend.

As so often has been the case, nature provides the answer with a little help from science!

Hemp Extract is the legal, non-psychoactive form of the cannabis sativa plant.

Since this can be such a confusing topic, it is important to understand the names and terminologies. Therefore, for simplicity's sake, Hemp Extract will be used when referring to cannabidiol or CBD throughout this book. Hemp Extract is the legal, non-psychoactive form of the cannabis sativa plant.

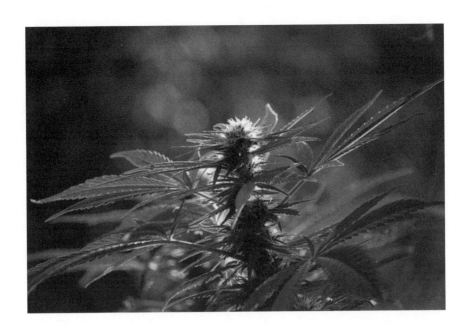

"A wise man ought to realize that health

is his most valuable possession."

-Hippocrates

CHAPTER 2: HEMP — A MUCH MISUNDERSTOOD PLANT

Knowledge about the many important uses of the hemp plant (also known as cannabis) has been around for millennia. Carbon tests have discovered that the Chinese were using hemp fiber for weaving as far back as 8000 BC. Evidence points to the fact that it was probably the earliest plant cultivated for textile fiber.

The cultivation of hemp spread throughout the ancient world. In addition to China, India, Greece, Africa and Europe, it was used in Egypt and other Middle Eastern countries. References to the plant show up on ancient Mesopotamian cuneiform tablets and in Egyptian hieroglyphics on palace and tomb walls.

Hemp has been cultivated in Great Britain since 800 AD. It was a necessary raw material that had many important uses. Henry VIII told farmers to plant hemp to supply the fiber to make fabric, riggings, sails and pennants for the Royal Navy. Hemp was the raw material that was turned into paper for making maps and books.

The Spaniards first introduced hemp as fiber to the New World in 1545. Colonial America quickly became reliant on the growing of hemp. In the 1700s, King James I ordered every colonist to grow 100 hemp plants, specifically for export.

Our founding fathers considered hemp to be economically important to the new country. Many of our founding fathers, including George Washington, were hemp enthusiasts. Thomas Jefferson also grew the hemp fiber as a primary cash crop and commented, "Hemp is of the first necessity to the wealth and protection of the country."

Hemp played a major role in American economic prosperity for hundreds of years. The 1850 U.S. census documented approximately 8,400 hemp plantations of at least 2,000 acres.

Hemp was considered so important in our early history that it was acknowledged as legal tender. For over 200 years colonial America used the hemp plant as an approved currency for tax payment.

Hemp as Medicine

The medicinal properties of hemp were also known in our ancient past. The first recorded medical use was described in Indo-Chinese medical texts more than 5,000 years ago. They described how it could be used for a variety of physical and mental conditions.

According to Chinese legend, in 2737 BC Emperor Shen Neng was one of the first major leaders in the ancient world to officially prescribe cannabis tea to treat various illnesses — including gout, rheumatism, malaria, and poor memory.

The medicinal use of the hemp plant spread throughout the Greek and Roman empires and then to the Islamic empire. During the Middle Ages, it was used as a topical salve to alleviate muscle and joint pain.

Although the agricultural use of hemp fiber in the United States was known for hundreds of years, it wasn't until 1839 when its medicinal properties were recognized.

An Irish medical doctor, William B. O'Shaughnessy, was the person responsible for enlightening the American medical profession to the healing properties of hemp. He had served many years in India as a doctor in the British East India Company and brought his extensive knowledge of the medicinal uses of hemp back with him. Dr. O'Shaughnessy passionately shared the healing benefits of hemp with his medical colleagues. Insomnia, pain, muscle spasms and other physical conditions were just a few of the numerous conditions he wrote about.

In 1851, hemp was added to the U.S. Pharmacopeia, an official public standard for all prescriptions and over-the-counter medications. It listed the medicinal benefits as treatment for many conditions, including neuralgia, tetanus, typhus, cholera, rabies, dysentery, alcoholism, opiate addiction, anthrax, leprosy, incontinence, gout, convulsive disorders, tonsillitis, insanity, excessive menstrual bleeding, and uterine bleeding.

Hemp became a common ingredient in many medical formulations. By the early 1900s, hemp was the second most common ingredient in medications. There were more than 2,000 preparations containing hemp from over 280 manufacturers. At that time, pharmaceutical companies such as Eli Lilly, Wyeth, Park-Davis, Sharp and Dohme were all making medicinal hemp formulations.

The 20th Century – The Dark Ages for Hemp

By the early 1900s agricultural hemp had become a major cash crop throughout the entire U.S. The medicinal uses of Hemp Extract were embraced by the medical profession and the public alike. However, there were sinister forces at play that would eventually alter the course of the hemp story for the next 70 years.

There are many explanations and theories as to why the government outlawed hemp. But the end result was the demise of farming agricultural hemp and the many industries that were reliant upon it. Hemp, thus, became a contraband crop as well as an illegal ingredient in medicinal formulas.

The most substantiated explanation for the demise of the hemp industry revolves around corporate greed and government collusion.

By the 1930s the hemp industry was a booming business. New machinery, which separated the fiber from the rest of the plant, had been invented and was affordable. These innovations simplified the harvesting and production. Growing hemp became very cost-effective.

Manufacturers were also interested in byproducts such as the seed oil for paint and lacquer, and the fiber for paper and cloth. According to the February 1938 issue of *Popular Mechanics*, hemp was then on the verge of becoming "the billion-dollar crop."

As it turns out, what was a boom for some would become a threat to others.

Around that time, there was a convergence of several major companies who conspired to destroy the hemp industry, which included the new petroleum-based synthetic textile companies. The 1930s saw DuPont patenting their new "plastic fiber." DuPont petrochemical company was making cellophane, nylon and Dacron from fossil fuels. DuPont held the patents on many synthetics and became a leader in the development of paint, rayon, synthetic rubber, plastics, chemicals, photographic film, insecticides and agricultural chemicals. Hemp was in competition with many of these new petroleum-based products.

Another major player in this drama was William Randolph Hearst. He was a powerful newspaper and lumber baron who saw hemp as the biggest threat to his businesses. Hearst had vast timber holdings that were to supply the raw material for his paper company. He planned to take over the paper industry with his low-quality paper. However, his grand plans were threatened by the hemp industry, which was able to produce low-cost, high-quality paper.

Powerful industrialist DuPont and media baron Hearst, as well as other senior government cronies, decided to band together. They planned a powerful propaganda campaign to demonize agricultural hemp with the intention of stopping all hemp production and removing it from the marketplace.

Under the influence of lobbying efforts by DuPont, Hearst and several other powerful groups, in September 1937 the U.S. government enacted prohibitive tax laws against the growing of hemp. Later that year hemp production was banned altogether.

In that same year, DuPont filed its patent on nylon, a synthetic fiber that took over many of the textile and rope markets that would have gone to hemp.

At that time, GM built more than half the American cars on the road. With hemp products now unavailable, GM turned to DuPont. This now guaranteed DuPont a captive market for paints, varnishes, plastics, and rubber, all of which could have been made from hemp. Furthermore, all GM cars would subsequently be designed to use tetra-ethyl leaded fuel exclusively, containing additives that DuPont manufactured.

Despite the regulations and restrictions, the prescription of medical hemp for medicinal use remained legal until 1970. At that time the federal government enacted the Comprehensive Drug Abuse Prevention and Control Act (now know as the Federal Controlled

Substance Act). Hemp was categorized as a Schedule 1 controlled substance, making it illegal for physicians to prescribe any hemp formulas to their patients.

As a result of these new laws, hemp all but disappeared from the American scene. The many benefits derived from the hemp plant were denied to American citizens.

The good news is that a hemp renaissance is now under way!

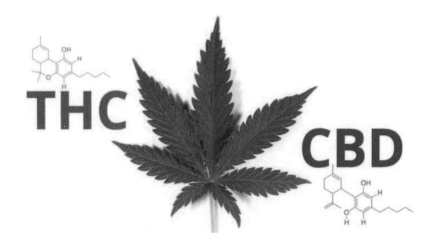

"Cannabis is the single most versatile herbal remedy, and the most useful plant on Earth. No other single plant contains as wide a range of medically active herbal constituents."

- *Dr. Ethan Russo, Neurologist and Medical Scientist*

CHAPTER 3: LET'S UNRAVEL THE HEMP EXTRACT VS. MARIJUANA CONFUSION

Understanding why the hemp plant is such a powerful healing medicine requires some explanation and important distinctions. Unfortunately, there is a great deal of confusion and misunderstanding about this subject. This is partially because we have been taught that all cannabis plants were psychoactive and mood altering, and partially because there are so many new discoveries that have not yet entered into mainstream awareness.

The purpose of this chapter is to help you understand the correct terminology and the distinct differences between what is known as agricultural hemp and marijuana, the psychoactive form or variety of cannabis. It will also eliminate any concerns you may have that the active ingredients in hemp, known as cannabidiol or Hemp Extract, are in any way illegal or harmful.

The hemp plant is a plant species called cannabis sativa. The hemp plant and the cannabis sativa plant are different names for the same plant.

All cannabis plants contain unique compounds called cannabinoids. One type of cannabinoids is called cannabidiol, or Hemp Extract. It is oil found in the cannabis sativa plant that has no psychoactive or euphoric effects. It is especially prevalent in the flowers and buds, and, to a lesser degree, in the stems and stalks of the plant.

The name cannabidiol, or CBD, can also be referred to as Hemp Extract.

Hemp Extract is just one of the 144 oils that can be found in the cannabis plant. Hemp Extract is found in the highest percentage of all the cannabinoid compounds contained in the cannabis plant. While cannabis also contains other compounds such as terpenes (chemicals that produce fragrances), vitamins, mineral, proteins and chlorophyll, the cannabinoids are the most important.

What Is THC?

One of the other oils found in the cannabis plant is known as THC (tetrahydrocannabinol). This is the oil that when ingested will initiate the "high" or euphoric feeling associated with marijuana.

The cannabis plant has been bred over time to have different ratios of oils in them. Those plants with high THC and low Hemp Extract oils were used more for recreational purposes. These were the cannabis sativa plants that have been selectively bred to have very high amounts of THC and low amounts of Hemp Extract.

Other cannabis plants have been bred to have high amounts of Hemp Extract and very low amounts of THC. This strain has many medicinal properties but will not create a feeling of euphoria or getting "high."

When Hemp Extract has less than 0.3% THC by weight, it is considered a dietary supplement. It is also now legal to be sold over the counter in all 50 states.

More than 23,000 studies worldwide have validated that the bioactive components of the hemp plant address many health conditions. It is important to emphasize this fact. If a strain of the cannabis sativa plant has been bred to have more than 0.3% by weight of THC, it is considered marijuana. This plant will cause you to get "high" because it has psychoactive effects. It also has many medicinal benefits. However, it is still an illegal Schedule 1 drug in many states.

To date there are 29 states and the District of Columbia that have legalized marijuana for strictly medicinal purposes. Some have also legalized it for recreational use as well.

Hemp Extract Has No Psychoactive Effects

To make this point perfectly clear, if the strain of cannabis sativa plant has been bred to have less than 0.3% of TCH in weight, it is classified by the government as legal for over-the-counter sales. This form of cannabis is called Hemp Extract.

According to Dan Sutton of Tantalus Labs, a Canadian company that specializes in cannabis cultivation technology, "the core agricultural differences between medical cannabis and hemp are largely in their genetic parentage and cultivation environment."

A special CNN report stated, "CBD oil from industrial hemp is already legal in all 50 states because the initial product, hemp, contains no traceable amounts of THC, and therefore is already legal to transport across state lines. Industrial hemp is genetically bred to have high levels of CBD, which is non-psychoactive, and safe for children and the elderly to consume (there is no 'high')." http:// ireport.cnn.com/docs/DOC-1251365

All the information in this book will be about the legal form of hemp that has been thoroughly tested for low THC (0.3%) and high amounts of cannabidiol (Hemp Extract) from the cannabis sativa plant.

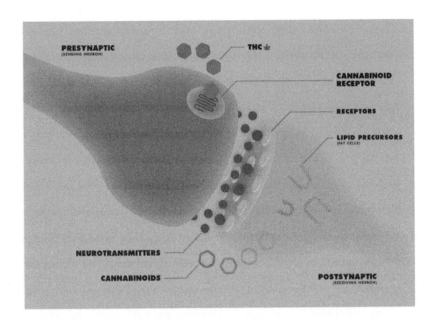

"The endogenous cannabinoid system is one of the most important physiologic systems involved in establishing and maintaining human health."

-*Bradley E. Alger, Ph.D.,* professor emeritus in the

Department of Physiology at the University of Maryland School of Medicine

CHAPTER 4: IT'S TIME TO MEET YOUR AMAZING ENDOCANNABINOID SYSTEM

Never heard of the endocannabinoid system before? Don't worry, you are not alone! In fact, it would be safe to say that 99% of Americans have yet to be introduced to this important system that plays a major role in maintaining your health.

There is a growing awareness and interest among scientists and medical practitioners about this relatively recent discovery. The endocannabinoid system (ECS) deserves lots of attention because it has been recognized as one of the most fundamental physiological systems inherent in our body for creating and supporting optimal health.

We have Dr. Raphael Mechoulam to thank for this groundbreaking discovery. Dr. Mechoulam, an Israeli organic chemist, professor of Medicinal Chemistry at the Hebrew University of Jerusalem, and pioneer in the field of cannabis research, is considered one of the giants of cannabis research. For the past 50 years, he and his team have succeeded in discovering the major plant cannabinoids in the cannabis plant, THC (tetrahydrocannabinol) and Hemp Extract (cannabidiol).

The ability to isolate these cannabinoids was the first stepping-stone to the discovery of another major breakthrough, the existence of our endocannabinoid system. The ECS is acknowledged as one of the most significant discoveries of our time.

According to Dr. Mechoulam, "By using a plant that has been around for thousands of years, we discovered a new physiological system of immense importance. We wouldn't have been able to get there if we had not looked at the plant."

Why is there such excitement among scientists and health practitioners? **It turns out that the ECS is a primordial language that nerves and brain cells use to communicate. From womb to tomb, across countless generations, the endocannabinoid system guides and protects all vital physiological processes.**

The discovery of the endocannabinoid system has breathtaking implications for nearly every area of medicine, including reproductive biology. Dr. Mauro Maccarrone at the University of Teramo, Italy, describes the endocannabinoid system as the "guardian angel" or "gatekeeper" of mammalian reproduction, with the endocannabinoid signaling system controlling the reproduction process – governing spermatogenesis, fertilization, transport of the zygote through the oviduct, implantation, and fetal development.

The Ancient History of the Endocannabinoid System

While the endocannabinoid system has only just recently made its debut onto the scientific stage, it is actually a very ancient system that has existed within all animal life forms except insects.

Due to the presence of cannabinoid receptor-like proteins in nematodes and sea squirts, it is speculated that the ECS began evolving 600 million years ago. The ECS and its receptors exist in fish, reptiles, earthworms, leeches, amphibians, birds and mammals.

With its long evolutionary history, scientists realized that the ECS had to have served an important and basic function in animal physiology.

What's the Big Deal About the Endocannabinoid System?

The ECS is possibly the single most important system within our entire body. It is responsible for maintaining a process called homeostasis. Basically, if our ECS is out of whack, the health of our entire body could be at risk.

There is one biological principle that is essential for maintaining a healthy functioning body. That principle is called homeostasis.

Homeostasis means that biological systems are actively regulated to maintain conditions within a narrow, healthy range. The intelligence of the body ensures that critical functions are always in proper balance. For instance, our body doesn't want its temperature to be too hot or too cold, or blood sugar levels too high or too low. Conditions need to be *just right* for our cells to be functioning optimally. Without this perfect, rather narrow range of regulation, we would die.

As it turns out, that is exactly the job of the ECS. It is a vital molecular system for helping to maintain homeostasis—it ensures that cells stay in their "Goldilocks" zone of "just right" at all times.

Another way to understand homeostasis is to imagine a traffic cop directing traffic at a very busy intersection. The task is to seamlessly direct and manage a smooth flow of traffic in all directions. His skilled management of the flow prevents bottlenecks, collisions and chaos. That is exactly the job of the ECS. It takes on the role of a traffic cop to all the major systems of the body, such as the immune system, respiratory system, nervous system, reproductive system, etc.

The ECS ensures that the communication between all the biological systems is working perfectly. Some of the processes the ECS controls include pain perception, gastrointestinal motility, memory, sleep, response to stress, anxiety, depression, bone repair, growth of new brain cells, reduction of excessive inflammation, regulation of hormonal systems, fertility, and protection from strokes and other neurodegenerative problems.

Researchers from all parts of the world have come to acknowledge the vast medical potential of the ECS. Summarized in a 2006 review by the National Institutes of Health (NIH):

"In the past decade, the endocannabinoid system has been implicated in a growing number of physiological functions, both in the central and peripheral nervous systems and in peripheral organs... modulating the activity of the endocannabinoid system turned out to hold therapeutic promise in a wide range of disparate diseases and pathological conditions, ranging from mood and anxiety disorders, movement disorders such as Parkinson's and Huntington's disease, neuropathic pain, multiple sclerosis and spinal cord injury, to cancer, atherosclerosis, myocardial infarction, stroke, hypertension, glaucoma, obesity/metabolic syndrome, and osteoporosis, to name just a few…"

The ECS regulates the homeostasis of the following functions:

Appetite

Metabolism

Pain

Sleep

Mood

Movement

Temperature

Memory and learning

Immune function

Inflammation

Neural development

Neuroprotection

Cardiovascular function

Digestion

Reproduction

This is why the ECS is such a big deal! Every important physiological function of our body is regulated and kept in balance by a properly functioning ECS.

CBDs and Your Endocannabinoid System

Dr. Mechoulam first discovered the endocannabinoid system while trying to understand the effects of the cannabinoid molecules, and thus named it the endocannabinoid system for this reason.

Cannabinoids are the chemical molecules that communicate with the ECS. They provide vital nutrients necessary for the normal functioning of the human body and the prevention of disease.

There are two types of cannabinoid molecules:

- One type is referred to as *endogenous,* which means our own body naturally makes it. These molecules interact with cannabinoid receptors on the membranes of the cells to regulate basic functions including mood, memory, appetite, pain, sleep and many more.

- The other type of cannabinoids is *exogenous,* meaning they originate from outside the body. The cannabinoids found in marijuana, such as tetrahydrocannabinol (THC), and those from the cannabis plant, called cannabidiol (CBD), are considered exogenous, or coming from the outside.

When the exogenous cannabinoids are ingested, they interact with endogenous cannabinoid receptors to produce physical and psychological effects in the body. They can also regulate basic functions such as mood, memory, appetite, pain, sleep, etc.

In order to have an effect on the body, the cannabinoid molecules must first dock into docking stations on the membranes of each cell, called receptor sites.

Cannabinoid receptors are present throughout the body, embedded in cell membranes, and are believed to be more numerous than any other receptor system. Also, they function as subtle sensing devices, tiny vibrating scanners perpetually primed to pick up biochemical cues that flow through fluids surrounding each cell.

The ECS has two types of receptors: CB1 and CB2. Each receptor responds to different cannabinoids, but some cannabinoids can interact with both.

CB1 receptors are found throughout the body, but are mostly present in the brain and spinal cord. For example, there are CB1 receptors in the hypothalamus, which are involved with appetite regulation, and the amygdala, which plays a role in memory and emotional processing. CB1 receptors are also found in nerve endings, where they act to reduce sensations of pain.

CB2 receptors tend to be found in the peripheral nervous system. They are especially concentrated in immune cells. When CB2 receptors are activated, they work to regulate immunity and reduce inflammation, which play a role in many diseases.

CB2 receptors are also present in the gut, spleen, liver, heart, kidneys, bones, blood vessels, lymph cells, endocrine glands and reproductive organs.

The CB2 receptors regulate the cells of the immune system, i.e., monocytes, macrophages, B-cells, T-cells and thymus gland cells. They are involved with swelling from injuries, immune response, cell migration and programmed cell death. When activated, they have an anti-inflammatory effect.

Hemp Extract works its healing effect by indirectly increasing the activity of CB2 receptors. Hemp Extract signals the body to increase more of its endogenous cannabinoids. Hemp Extract can also activate other receptors in the body's system that have to do with pain, perception and inflammation.

However, the ECS is a very complicated system. For instance, many tissues contain both CB1 and CB2 receptors, each linked to a different action. This helps to explain why Hemp Extract can successfully alleviate so many varied health conditions.

Health Is All About Balance

Whether the result of poor diet, lack of exercise, drug abuse, physical or emotional stress, environmental toxins or genetic factors, endocannabinoid deficits are associated with a reduced ability or inability to adapt to chronic stress. Prolonged exposure to these numerous stressors will eventually deplete the proper endocannabinoid response, also known as endocannabinoid tone. This, in turn, has an adverse impact on many physiological processes.

Stress of any kind can knock the body's delicate homeostasis process out of balance. These delicate feedback loops are impaired. Imagine what happens when the traffic lights are out at a busy intersection. Total chaos ensues, along with car wrecks and injuries!

An endocannabinoid deficiency will also create chaos to the many regulating systems of the body. This is when Hemp Extract can come to the rescue. When our ECS is overwhelmed by so many stressful insults, the body needs extra support and protection. Ongoing research has shown how effective Hemp Extract supplementation can be. **Hemp Extract has the amazing ability to safely and effectively restore homeostasis throughout our body.**

There is a growing list of conditions that Hemp Extract has proven to help. A partial list includes migraines, fibromyalgia, psychiatric conditions, irritable bowel disease, seizures, brain damage, autoimmune issues and chronic pain.

Why Are Hemp Extracts Important for You?

Hemp Extract assists with maintaining homeostasis within the body. Homeostasis is so important that most chronic diseases are regarded as a result of its disturbance. As we get older, the body's internal environment becomes progressively less stable. As a result, we are more vulnerable to illness.

If we take into account the amount of stress that most of us are under in a normal day, as well as the lack of good nutrition in the average diet, it's no wonder that we are experiencing unprecedented levels of diabetes, obesity, autism, anxiety, autoimmune conditions, and other expressions of imbalance.

Hemp Extract delivers a wide range of benefits of its own, which can figure into helping our ECS maintain an existing state of wellness as well as addressing a state of imbalance.

It's also important to know that Hemp Extracts are not just about helping to regain and ensure optimal health. Hemp Extracts should also be recognized as playing a major role for achieving optimal wellness as well as contributing to an effective anti-aging program.

As a result of these wide-ranging effects, many researchers now believe that Hemp Extract may be the single most important cannabinoid ever discovered.

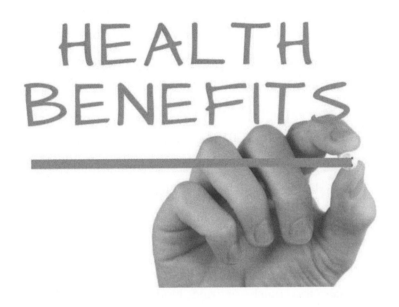

HEALTH
BENEFITS

"There were never so many able, active minds at work on the problems of disease as now, and all their discoveries are tending toward the simple truth that you can't improve on nature."

-Thomas Edison

CHAPTER 5: HEMP EXTRACT USES A TO Z

Acne

Acne is a common skin disease characterized by elevated sebum production and inflammation of the sebaceous glands. It is a condition that affects people of all ages, from puberty on. However, teenagers and young adults suffer from acne the most, caused by hormonal changes experienced during puberty. Acne is very visible, leading to psychological issues like anxiety and depression.

One of the causes of acne is the overproduction of sebum, which is an oily substance that maintains the condition of the skin. Hemp Extract has the ability to block the stimulation of sebum production and reduce inflammation.

A study conducted in 2010 by a Hungarian scientist, Dr. Tamas Biro, intended to analyze the impact of Hemp Extract on the skin. He isolated skin cells and applied Hemp Extract, to check how the cannabinoid interacts with our own endocannabinoids. The findings revealed that the endocannabinoid cells play an important role in determining how much oil the skin produces. When our body produces too much of one kind of a neurotransmitter called *anandamide,* which is part of the ECS, it produces a surge of oil.

On the other hand, inadequate anandamide will result in dryness and skin diseases such as eczema. When Dr. Biro administered Hemp Extract on the skin cells, anandamide was reduced and oil production was halted.

A recent study published in 2014 used Hemp Extract on sebaceous glands, which secrete oily sebum, causing acne. The researchers stated that Hemp Extract worked as a "highly effective" drug or product that causes drying out of the sebaceous glands.

They also found that Hemp Extract inhibited both lipogenic action (the way the body converts energy to fat for storage), and the production of sebocytes (cells in the sebaceous glands which produce the oil which coats the hair and skin of mammals). Both processes are known to contribute to acne.

The study concluded: "Collectively, our findings suggest that, due to the combined lipostatic, anti-proliferative and anti-inflammatory effects, Hemp Extract has potential as a promising therapeutic agent for the treatment of acne vulgaris."

It is recommended to use Hemp Extract orally as well as topically for best results.

Pak J Pharm Sci. 2015 Jul;28(4):1389-95.
The safety and efficacy of 3% Cannabis seeds extract cream for reduction of human cheek skin sebum and erythema content.

J Clin Invest. 2014 Sep;124(9):3713-24. doi: 10.1172/JCI64628. Epub 2014 Jul 25.
Cannabidiol exerts sebostatic and anti-inflammatory effects on human sebocytes.

Trends Pharmacol Sci. 2009 Aug;30(8):411-20. doi: 10.1016/j.tips. 2009.05.004. Epub 2009 Jul 14.
The endocannabinoid system of the skin in health and disease: novel perspectives and therapeutic opportunities.

Exp Dermatol. 2016 Sep;25(9):701-7. doi: 10.1111/exd.13042. Epub 2016 Jun 15.
Differential effectiveness of selected non-psychotropic phytocannabinoids on human sebocyte functions implicates their introduction in dry/seborrhoeic skin and acne treatment.

Addictions/Alcoholism and Other Substance Addictions

Substance addictions are hard to kick. Whether the addition is to alcohol, tobacco, heroin, cocaine, amphetamine or the psychoactive marijuana, there a strong physiological as well emotional desire to return to the preferred substance.

The American Society of Disease Medicine characterizes addiction as "an inability to consistently abstain, impairment in behavioral control, and craving, diminished recognition of significant problems with one's behaviors and interpersonal relationships, and a dysfunctional emotional response. Like other chronic diseases, addiction often involves cycles of relapse and remission. Without treatment or engagement in recovery activities, addiction is progressive and can result in disability or premature death."

The use of Hemp Extract has shown that it helped reduce the physical cravings as well as accompanying feelings of anxiety and depression.

In a double-blind, placebo-controlled study, heroin addicts were administered a single dose of Hemp Extract over three consecutive days. Their propensity for craving was then tested compared to the placebo. The subjects taking Hemp Extract found their cravings were lessened, an effect that lasted for seven days after treatment.

This essentially means that the effect of Hemp Extract on the addict's brain initiated a kind of rewiring that may reduce craving and relapse on a more long-term basis.

Similar findings were observed in cigarette smokers. They were given an inhaler containing Hemp Extract. The results showed that they smoked 40% fewer cigarettes, compared to a placebo group where there was no change.

The authors noted, "We found that Hemp Extract seems to reduce the salience of cues. It also can reduce anxiety and may affect a memory process called 'reconsolidation,' which is when a memory of the reward of smoking is re-activated by seeing someone smoking, and it is rendered vulnerable to destruction."

Whatever the addiction may be, the use of Hemp Extract is proving to be a valuable tool in helping to free people from their addictive cravings. This includes heroin, tobacco, alcohol, marijuana and cocaine.

Molecular Psychiatry (2003) 8, 373–382. doi:10.1038/sj.mp.4001269
Glutamatergic mechanisms in addiction

Neurotherapeutics. 2015 Oct; 12(4): 807–815.
Published online 2015 Aug 13. doi: 10.1007/s13311-015-0373-7
PMCID: PMC4604178
Early Phase in the Development of Cannabidiol as a Treatment for Addiction: Opioid Relapse Takes Initial Center Stage

Addict Behav. 2013 Sep;38(9):2433-6. doi: 10.1016/j.addbeh.
2013.03.011. Epub 2013 Apr 1.

Cannabidiol reduces cigarette consumption in tobacco smokers: preliminary findings.

Addict Biol. 2013 Mar;18(2):286-96. doi: 10.1111/j. 1369-1600.2012.00483.x. Epub 2012 Aug 2. Cannabidiol inhibits the reward-facilitating effect of morphine: involvement of 5-HT1A receptors in the dorsal raphe nucleus.

J Clin Pharm Ther. 2013 Apr;38(2):162-4. doi: 10.1111/jcpt.12018. Epub 2012 Oct 24. Cannabidiol for the treatment of cannabis withdrawal syndrome: a case report

Br J Pharmacol. 2017 Oct;174(19):3242-3256. doi: 10.1111/bph. 13724. Epub 2017 Mar 9. Cannabidiol regulation of emotion and emotional memory processing: relevance for treating anxiety-related and substance abuse disorders.

ADHD

ADHD, or Attention Deficit Hyperactivity Disorder, is a controversial diagnosis indicated by hyperactivity, impulsivity, and distractibility. It affects children as well as adults. People with ADHD have difficulties with focus, attention and concentration.

A study published in the *Journal of Substance Use and Misuse* showed that people who have used Hemp Extract were helped in the management of impulsive and hyperactive behaviors. This led researchers to suggest that Hemp Extract can help in the therapeutic aid of those with ADHD.

Additional published research studied the effect of Hemp Extract on 30 patients that did not respond to Ritalin or Adderall. The majority of the subjects experienced improvement in sleep and concentration as well as reduced impulsivity.

Scientists have associated ADHD with clinical endocannabinoid deficiency. Persons with this deficiency have slowed-down neurotransmitter speed, and their brains need more time to focus and concentrate.

According to researchers, standard medications are more demanding on patients, while Hemp Extract brings control that enables them to work, love, and live without feeling intoxicated.

Hemp Extract is a welcome alternative solution used to increase focus and attention without drug inducing side effects. It is actually safely addressing an underlying problem, ECS deficiency.

Clin Nucl Med. 2014 Feb;39(2):e129-34. doi: 10.1097/RLU. 0b013e31829f9119.
Searching for a neurobiological basis for self-medication theory in ADHD comorbid with substance use disorders: an in vivo study of dopamine transporters using (99m)Tc-TRODAT-1 SPECT.

J Psychopharmacol. 2012 Oct;26(10):1317-32. doi: 10.1177/0269881112441865. Epub 2012 Apr 9.
Cannabidiol and clozapine reverse MK-801-induced deficits in social interaction and hyperactivity in Sprague-Dawley rats.

Drug Alcohol Depend. 2014 Feb 1;135:88-94. doi: 10.1016/ j.drugalcdep.2013.11.013. Epub 2013 Nov 25.

Childhood and current ADHD symptom dimensions are associated with more severe cannabis outcomes in college students.

Psychiatry Res. 2012 Dec 30;200(2-3):581-7. doi: 10.1016/j.psychres. 2012.06.003. Epub 2012 Jul 4.
Neuropsychological performance, impulsivity, ADHD symptoms, and novelty seeking in compulsive buying disorder.

Amyotrophic lateral sclerosis (ALS)

Amyotrophic lateral sclerosis (ALS) is considered a fatal neurodegenerative disease of the motor neuron system with limited therapeutic options. ALS destroys nerve cells that control muscles. Patients progressively experience weakness that hinders movement, speech, swallowing and breathing.

In studies on ALS, mouse models were given a daily dose of either THC, cannabidiol, cannabidiol plus THC, or a placebo following the onset of signs of the disease. Results showed that among these options, Hemp Extract was most effective in delaying the progression of the disease.

Scientists said research from California Pacific Medical Center in San Francisco showed that the FDA-approved drug for ALS, riluzole, extends life on average by about two months, while evidence from their study suggests that a hemp-based therapy could have a much greater effect, perhaps extending life by three years or more. This significant finding is a profound discovery, offering hope to ALS patients.

Neuropharmacology. 2017 Sep 15;124:157-169. doi: 10.1016/
j.neuropharm.2017.03.037. Epub 2017 Mar 31.
Evaluation of monoacylglycerol lipase as a therapeutic target in a
transgenic mouse model of ALS.

Neuropharmacology. 2015 Apr;91:148-56. doi: 10.1016/
j.neuropharm.2014.12.001. Epub 2014 Dec 12.
Comparative biochemical characterization of the monoacylglycerol
lipase inhibitor KML29 in brain, spinal cord, liver, spleen, fat and
muscle tissue.

Am J Hosp Palliat Care. 2010 Aug;27(5):347-56. doi:
10.1177/1049909110369531. Epub 2010 May 3.
Cannabis and amyotrophic lateral sclerosis: hypothetical and practical
applications, and a call for clinical trials.

Alzheimer's Disease

Alzheimer's disease is a progressive type of dementia that destroys
memory, behavior and thinking. The disease causes brain cells to
degenerate and die, resulting in a steady decline in memory,
intellectual and social skills. As brain cells die, the brain also shrinks.

Scientists believe Alzheimer's disease is caused by a combination of
genetic, lifestyle and environmental factors. Age seems to play a role,
as risk increases significantly at and beyond the age of 65. The
disease affects nearly half of people over the age of 85. An
estimated 5.5 million Americans are living with Alzheimer's.

The prevailing theory has been a build-up of amyloid plaque.
Medications that have targeted that theory have essentially failed to
produce any significant effect.

A new theory has emerged as to the underlying cause of Alzheimer's. Research from Harvard has shown that as you age your mitochondria tend to malfunction. The DNA in aging mitochondria is harmfully altered by mutations, and the mitochondria produce destructive free radicals whose oxidative activity destroys neurons.

Strategies targeting inflammation, oxidative stress and impaired glucose uptake (the food for the brain) are producing the greatest possibilities for halting the progression and even reversing the symptoms.

Hemp Extract has shown to possess neuroprotective, anti-inflammatory, and antioxidant properties in vitro. These properties suggest that the compound could be therapeutically beneficial for reducing or even inhibiting the cognitive and functional impairment that occurs with Alzheimer's disease.

The CB2 cannabinoid found in Hemp Extract can down-regulate expression by pro-inflammatory cytokines-associated transcription factors, alleviate inflammation of neurons, and promote protection of the neurons.

Hemp Extract stimulates CB2 receptors in the immune cells in the brain. This results in a decreased inflammatory response. So long-term use of Hemp Extract would decrease the extent of damage caused by the inflammation.

Findings also indicate that Hemp Extract promotes neurogenesis, or the growth and development of new brain cells. This is a really exciting discovery. Creating new brain cells helps to reduce the deterioration of cognitive functions. In addition, it improves psychomotor agitation, aggression and communication.

Understanding the real cause of Alzheimer's and dementia is an important discovery in the understanding of Alzheimer's disease as well as for its treatment and prevention.

While it requires a multi-pronged approach, which includes diet, lifestyle, and targeted supplementation, Hemp Extract is certainly proving to be a significant piece of this challenging puzzle.

CNS Drugs. 2015 Aug;29(8):615-23. doi: 10.1007/s40263-015-0270-y.
Cannabinoids for the Treatment of Agitation and Aggression in Alzheimer's Disease.

Biochem Soc Trans. 2013 Dec;41(6):1583-7. doi: 10.1042/BST20130140.
Endocannabinoid signaling in Alzheimer's disease.

J Neurochem. 2004 Apr;89(1):134-41.
Neuroprotective effect of cannabidiol, a non-psychoactive component from Cannabis sativa, on beta-amyloid-induced toxicity in PC12 cells.

J Alzheimers Dis. 2015;43(4):1115-36. doi: 10.3233/JAD-141635.
The role of endocannabinoid signaling in the molecular mechanisms of neurodegeneration in Alzheimer's disease.

CNS Neurosci Ther. 2009 Winter;15(1):65-75. doi: 10.1111/j.1755-5949.2008.00065.x.
Cannabidiol: a promising drug for neurodegenerative disorders?

Curr Pharm Des. 2008;14(23):2299-3305.
The role of the endocannabinoid system in Alzheimer's disease: facts and hypotheses.

Phytother Res. 2014 Jul;28(7):1007-13. doi: 10.1002/ptr.5095. Epub 2013 Nov 28.
Cannabidiol promotes amyloid precursor protein ubiquitination and reduction of beta amyloid expression in SHSY5YAPP+ cells through PPARγ involvement

Int. J. Mol. Sci. 2017, 18(1), 26; doi:10.3390/ijms18010026
Cannabidiol Modulates the Expression of Alzheimer's Disease-Related Genes in Mesenchymal Stem Cells

Front Pharmacol. 2017 Feb 3;8:20. doi: 10.3389/fphar.2017.00020. eCollection 2017.
In vivo Evidence for Therapeutic Properties of Cannabidiol (CBD) for Alzheimer's Disease.

CNS Neurol Disord Drug Targets. 2017;16(5):541-553. doi: 10.2174/1871527316666170413114210.
Neurological Aspects of Medical Use of Cannabidiol.

Anti-Aging Benefits

The science of anti-aging has proven that in order to ensure optimal health and wellbeing throughout your life, it is imperative to reduce inflammation and free-radical production, reduce stress and anxiety, improve sleep, create new brain cells, support a healthy immune system, and enhance insulin sensitivity.

Ongoing scientific research has shown that using Hemp Extract on a regular basis will support and enhance your body's ability to achieve all these key parameters of health. And the best news is that it is safe and effective.

You can consider Hemp Extract as a daily vitamin for keeping your body in homeostasis. Hemp Extract is proving to be a fountain of youth to ensure optimal wellness at any age!

Antibiotic Resistance

The widespread use of antibiotics for more than seven decades has created a very serious and unforeseen health crisis.

A recent report by Centers for Disease Control (CDC) stated that around half of antibiotic prescriptions are not necessary. Another report from the World Health Organization (WHO) warned that the impact of such an overconsumption of antibiotics is catastrophic. Common bacteria are now evolving and generating resistance against a myriad of such commonly used antibiotics.

At least 2 million Americans are diagnosed with an antibiotic-resistant infection annually, and at least 23,000 people die every year as a result of antibiotic resistance.

The arsenal of antibiotics is proving less and less effective in combating antibiotic resistance.

This is of great concern. One of the most dangerous strains of resistant bacteria is called MRSA, short for methicillin-resistant Staphylococcus aurous. It is a bacterium that causes difficult-to-treat infections that are unresponsive to many antibiotics. Some strains are now immune to the most powerful last-resort antibiotic, vancomycin.

However, there is good news on the natural antibiotic front. British and Italian researchers have proven that Hemp Extract has a built-in capacity to fight against such drug-resistant bacteria. They discovered that the cannabinoids in Hemp Extract are as effective at killing the bugs as vancomycin and other antibiotics.

At least six such major resistant bacteria have been tested. In all the cases, Hemp Extract turned out to be much more effective against such antibiotic resistant bacteria than any other antibiotic.

Topical applications as well as oral use of Hemp Extract have shown to be very effective in specifically killing drug-resistant bacteria.

J Nat Prod. 2008 Aug;71(8):1427-30. doi: 10.1021/np8002673. Epub 2008 Aug 6.
Antibacterial cannabinoids from Cannabis sativa: a structure-activity study.

Antonie Van Leeuwenhoek. 1976;42(1-2):9-12.
Antibacterial activity of delta9-tetrahydrocannabinol and cannabidiol.
Cannabis plant extracts can effectively fight drug-resistant bacteria.
ABCNews.go.com/Technology/story?id=5787866&page=1

Anxiety

Anxiety-related disorders affect a huge segment of our population. It is estimated that 40 million people over the age of 18 experience some sort of anxiety.

Accumulating <u>evidence</u> from human experimental, clinical and epidemiological studies suggests that Hemp Extract has demonstrated powerful anti-anxiety properties.

Research has shown that not only is it safe and well-tolerated, but it is non-addictive and lacks the more dangerous side effects of the usual medications prescribed for anxiety disorders. It is helpful in treating the following anxiety-related disorders:

- Panic disorder
- Obsessive Compulsive Disorder (OCD)
- Social phobia
- Post-Traumatic Stress Disorder (PTSD)
- Generalized Anxiety Disorder (GAD)
- Mild to moderate depression

Hemp Extract exerts several actions in the brain that explain why it could be effective in treating anxiety. There are areas of the brain known to control emotional behavior, mood, sleep, stress, irritability, fear and even the sensation of "craving." Hemp Extract appears to attenuate the well-known "fight or flight" phenomenon to physical and mental stress, which reduces panic and anxiety behavior.

Research strongly supports Hemp Extract as a treatment for generalized anxiety disorder, panic disorder, social anxiety disorder, obsessive-compulsive disorder, and post-traumatic stress disorder.

Hemp Extract has clearly shown that it safely and effectively reduces feelings of fear and anxiety, while at the same time helping to restore a healthy stress response.

Rev Bras Psiquiatr. 2012 Jun;34 Suppl 1:S104-10.
Cannabidiol, a Cannabis sativa constituent, as an anxiolytic drug.
CNS Neurol Disord Drug Targets. 2014;13(6):953-60.
Antidepressant-like and anxiolytic-like effects of cannabidiol: a chemical compound of Cannabis sativa.

Neuropsychopharmacology. 2011 May;36(6):1219-26. doi: 10.1038/ npp.2011.6. Epub 2011 Feb 9.
Cannabidiol reduces the anxiety induced by simulated public speaking in treatment-naïve social phobia patients.

Neuropsychopharmacology. 2004 Feb;29(2):417-26.
Effects of cannabidiol (CBD) on regional cerebral blood flow.

CNS Drugs. 2013 Apr;27(4):301-19. doi: 10.1007/ s40263-013-0059-9.
Plant-based medicines for anxiety disorders, part 2: a review of clinical studies with supporting preclinical evidence.

Curr Top Med Chem. 2016;16(17):1924-42.
A Systematic Review of Plant-Derived Natural Compounds for Anxiety Disorders Vitam Horm. 2017;103:193-279. doi: 10.1016/ bs.vh.2016.09.006. Epub 2016 Nov 2.
The Endocannabinoid System and Anxiety.

Perm J. 2016 Fall;20(4):108-111. doi: 10.7812/TPP/16-005. Epub 2016 Oct 12.
Effectiveness of Cannabidiol Oil for Pediatric Anxiety and Insomnia as Part of Posttraumatic Stress Disorder: A Case Report.

Curr Top Med Chem. 2016;16(17):1924-42.
A Systematic Review of Plant-Derived Natural Compounds for Anxiety Disorders.

Arthritis – Osteoarthritis and Rheumatoid Arthritis

Arthritis is the inflammation of one or more joints, causing stiffness and pain in the tissues that surround the joints.

Arthritis is a term that actually refers to conditions of joint pain and joint disease. There are currently more than 100 types of arthritis, which include degenerative, inflammatory, autoimmune, infectious and metabolic.

Research has found that there are unusually high levels of CB2 receptors on the joint tissue of arthritis patients but not in healthy tissues. Hemp extract has shown to fight inflammation in the joints by activating the pathways of CB2 receptors. This is nature's way of reducing local inflammation.

Further research has shown that Hemp Extract is effective in both the prevention of joint damage and the treatment of arthritic conditions.

Hemp Extract also plays a role in immune system modulation, which means it helps in autoimmune conditions like rheumatoid arthritis.

The use of both oral and topical application of Hemp Extract is the most successful combination in reducing pain and helping to heal the damaged tissue of all forms of arthritis.

Rheumatology (Oxford). 2006 Jan;45(1):50-2. Epub 2005 Nov 9.
Preliminary assessment of the efficacy, tolerability and safety of a cannabis-based medicine (Sativex) in the treatment of pain caused by rheumatoid arthritis.

Proc Natl Acad Sci U S A. 2000 Aug 15;97(17):9561-6.

Eur J Neurosci. 2014 Feb;39(3):485-500. doi: 10.1111/ejn.12468.
Involvement of the endocannabinoid system in osteoarthritis pain.

Neurosci Lett. 2011 Aug 1;500(1):72-6. doi: 10.1016/j.neulet.
2011.06.004. Epub 2011 Jun 13.
The abnormal cannabidiol analogue O-1602 reduces nociception in a rat model of acute arthritis via the putative cannabinoid receptor GPR55.

J Psychopharmacol. 2011 Jan;25(1):121-30. doi:
10.1177/0269881110379283. Epub 2010 Sep 9.
Neural basis of anxiolytic effects of cannabidiol (CBD) in generalized social anxiety disorder: a preliminary report.

Pain. 2017 Sep 27. doi: 10.1097/j.pain.0000000000001052. [Epub ahead of print]
Attenuation of early phase inflammation by cannabidiol prevents pain and nerve damage in rat osteoarthritis.

Asthma

Asthma is a chronic respiratory disease that currently affects up to 25 million Americans. There are more than 4,000 deaths due to asthma each year.

Cannabinoid receptors have been found in lung tissue and are thought to play a vital role in the regulation of inflammation, muscular contractions and dilations, as well as other metabolic processes.

Early research suggests that Hemp Extract is an effective treatment for minimizing the inflammation experienced by so many asthma sufferers.

Another study found that Hemp Extract might influence a reduction in the major stimuli of mucus hyper-secretion, a prominent symptom experienced by those with asthma.

The research clearly shows that Hemp Extract is proving to be effective in addressing many of the factors of asthma. It acts as a bronchodilator, reduces inflammation in the lung, and reduces mucus production.

Curr Drug Targets. 2012 Jun;13(7):984-93.
The role of cannabinoids in inflammatory modulation of allergic respiratory disorders, inflammatory pain and ischemic stroke.

Clin Pharmacol Ther. 2011 Sep;90(3):388-91. doi: 10.1038/clpt.
2011.94. Epub 2011 Jun 29.
Allergen challenge increases anandamide in bronchoalveolar fluid of
patients with allergic asthma.

J Cell Mol Med. 2008 Dec;12(6A):2381-94. doi: 10.1111/j.
1582-4934.2008.00258.x. Epub 2008 Feb 4.
Activation of cannabinoid receptors prevents antigen-induced
asthma-like reaction in guinea pigs.

Int Arch Allergy Immunol. 2005 Sep;138(1):80-7. Epub 2005 Aug 11.
Endogenous cannabinoid receptor agonists inhibit neurogenic
inflammations in guinea pig airways.

Mediators of Inflammation
Volume 2015 (2015), Article ID 538670
Evaluation of Serum Cytokine Levels and the Role of Cannabidiol
Treatment in Animal Model of Asthma.

Autism Spectrum Disorder

Autism spectrum is a complex neurobehavioral disorder that includes
impairments in social language and communication skills. It is further
complicated by rigid, repetitive behaviors. ASD has a large variety of
symptoms and levels of impairment, with symptoms ranging from
minor limitations to overwhelming disabilities.

The use of Hemp Extract in the treatment of hypersensitivity to
physical sensations, noises and smells, as well as the hyperactivity
associated with the disorder, has shown promising results.

Research at the University of California confirmed the healing
properties of Hemp Extract. It showed that Hemp Extract works

against further brain function degradation and has evidence of powerful neuroprotective properties.

Hemp Extract has also been found to regulate emotion and focus specifically related to studies on autistic patients.

Israeli scientists have conducted clinical trials for Hemp Extract as a major cure for autistic children and teenagers. Hemp Extract is proving to be a very effective treatment.

There is mounting evidence that the use of Hemp Extract for children as well as adults is offering a safe and effective treatment for many of the symptoms and dysfunctions contributing to Autism Spectrum Disorder.

Neurotherapeutics
October 2015, Volume 12, Issue 4, pp 837–847 | Cite as
Endocannabinoid Signaling in Autism

J Autism Dev Disord. 2013 Nov;43(11):2686-95. doi: 10.1007/
s10803-013-1824-9.
Cannabinoid receptor type 2, but not type 1, is up-regulated in
peripheral blood mononuclear cells of children affected by autistic
disorders.

Curr Neuropharmacol. 2011 Mar;9(1):209-14. doi:
10.2174/157015911795017047.
Consequences of cannabinoid and monoaminergic system disruption
in a mouse model of autism spectrum disorders.

Brain Behav Immun. 2016 Nov;58:237-247. doi: 10.1016/j.bbi.
2016.07.152. Epub 2016 Jul 21.

Deficient adolescent social behavior following early-life inflammation is ameliorated by augmentation of anandamide signaling.

Parenting.com/news-break/cannabis-spray-treatment-helps-9-year-old-autism-learn-to-speak

Autoimmune Conditions

Autoimmune disorders affect up to 50 million Americans, with women being 75 percent of those affected. Although symptoms may vary greatly, all autoimmune diseases essentially result when inflammation initiates a response where the body attacks its own tissue.

Hemp Extract can benefit patients suffering autoimmune disorders because it activates a system of receptors that regulate inflammation and immune cell activity.

Hemp Extract helps to calm an overactive immune system, allowing the body's self-defense to return to homeostasis. Research has demonstrated that Hemp Extract can help the many autoimmune conditions. The specific autoimmune conditions that have been studied include rheumatoid arthritis, fibromyalgia, type 2 diabetes, celiac disease and inflammatory bowel diseases.

Since all autoimmune conditions involve an overactive immune system and chronic inflammation, it is only logical that the use of Hemp Extract would be beneficial for any kind of autoimmune issue.

Future Med Chem. Author manuscript; available in PMC 2010 Aug 1.
Published in final edited form as:
Future Med Chem. 2009 Oct; 1(7): 1333–1349.
doi: 10.4155/fmc.09.93
Cannabinoids as novel anti-inflammatory drugs.

J Neuroimmune Pharmacol. 2013 Dec;8(5):1265-76. doi: 10.1007/
s11481-013-9493-1. Epub 2013 Jul 28.
Cannabinoids decrease the th17 inflammatory autoimmune
phenotype.

Curr Opin Clin Nutr Metab Care. 2014 Mar;17(2):130-8. doi:
10.1097/MCO.0000000000000027.
The endocannabinoid system:
an emerging key player in inflammation.

Bone Health

Hemp Extract has demonstrated bone-healing and bone-building abilities. Studies have shown that the endocannabinoid system plays a significant role in growing, preserving and strengthening bones.

Thus, Hemp Extract can play a part in the prevention and treatment of osteoporosis.

A 2015 study found that cannabinoid receptors could trigger bone formation and strengthen the tissues that connect broken bones. Researchers found that bones treated with Hemp Extract healed faster and with a strengthened fracture callus. A "fracture callus" builds a natural bridge with cartilage between the areas of the break.

The cannabinoid system appears to regulate how much old bone material is broken down, how much fat is stored inside the bone, and how many new bone cells were allowed to be born.

Hemp Extract has one more important function when it comes to healthy bones: It stimulates bone-building cells to express the genes involved in producing the primary enzyme involved in bone healing.

Cannabidiol, a Major Non-Psychotropic Cannabis Constituent, Enhances Fracture Healing and Stimulates Lysyl Hydroxylase Activity in Osteoblasts
http://onlinelibrary.wiley.com/doi/10.1002/jbmr.2513/abstract;jsessionid=DBEF56DB42BCE5AEDD3BB6A9D3D0B03B.f03t02

Curr Neuropharmacol. 2010 Sep;8(3):243-53. doi: 10.2174/157015910792246173.
Cannabinoid receptors as target for treatment of osteoporosis: a tale of two therapies.

Calcif Tissue Int. 2010 Oct;87(4):285-97. doi: 10.1007/s00223-010-9378-8. Epub 2010 Jun 9.
Cannabinoids and bone: friend or foe?

Cell Metab. 2009 Aug;10(2):139-47. doi: 10.1016/j.cmet.2009.07.006.
Cannabinoid receptor type 1 protects against age-related osteoporosis by regulating osteoblast and adipocyte differentiation in marrow stromal cells.

Bone. 2011 May 1;48(5):997-1007. doi: 10.1016/j.bone.2011.01.001. Epub 2011 Jan 13.
The endovanilloid/endocannabinoid system: a new potential target for osteoporosis therapy.

J Neuroendocrinol. 2008 May;20 Suppl 1:69-74. doi: 10.1111/j.1365-2826.2008.01675.x.
Endocannabinoids and the regulation of bone metabolism.

Proc Natl Acad Sci U S A. 2006 Jan 17;103(3):696-701. Epub 2006 Jan 9.
Peripheral cannabinoid receptor, CB2, regulates bone mass.

Proc Natl Acad Sci U S A. 2006 Jan 17;103(3):696-701. Epub 2006 Jan 9.
Peripheral cannabinoid receptor, CB2, regulates bone mass.

Bipolar Disorder

Bipolar disorder is a complex mixture of different moods, causing dramatic mood swings and alternating between states of depression and mania.

Bipolar disorder can occur as a result of an imbalance of the endocannabinoid system. Since your ECS is scattered throughout the brain, it's only logical that it is involved in modulating many of the brain's functions, such as mood.

A dysfunctional ECS has been implicated in mood disorders such as bipolar disorder. Research has proven that Hemp Extract helps to restore the balance of our ECS and is even suggested to improve its function.

Investigation continues to validate that Hemp Extract has great potential as an effective and safe treatment of bipolar disorder symptoms by exerting antipsychotic, anticonvulsant and antianxiety effects.

J Psychopharmacol. 2005 May;19(3):293-300.
Cannabinoids in bipolar affective disorder: a review and discussion of their therapeutic potential.

J Psychopharmacol. 2010 Jan;24(1):135-7. doi: 10.1177/0269881108096521. Epub 2008 Sep 18.
Cannabidiol was ineffective for manic episode of bipolar affective disorder.

Cancer

Hemp Extract impacts cancer through several important mechanisms. It increases death of cancer cells through a mechanism of programmed cell suicide, known as *apoptosis*. This is only triggered in cancer cells.

One of the ways cancer grows is through angiogenesis, the formation of new blood vessels that supply the cancer cells with nutrients. A study has shown that Hemp Extract inhibits angiogenesis by multiple mechanisms.

Hemp Extract also helps fight cancer by reducing cancer cells' ability to migrate as well as adhere to and invade tissue, known as metastasis.

Hemp Extract not only helps to reduce inflammation, which is involved with cancer, but also reduces the ability of some types of tumor cells to reproduce.

Ongoing research with Hemp Extract shows that it is an effective modality that should be considered as part of a cancer protocol as well as supporting cancer prevention.

General Cancer Research

Br J Clin Pharmacol. 2013 Feb;75(2):303-12. doi: 10.1111/j. 1365-2125.2012.04298.x.
Cannabidiol as potential anticancer drug.

Br J Pharmacol. 2012 Nov;167(6):1218-31. doi: 10.1111/j. 1476-5381.2012.02050.x.
Cannabidiol inhibits angiogenesis by multiple mechanisms.

J Pain Symptom Manage. 2013 Apr;45(4):e1. doi: 10.1016/ j.jpainsymman.2013.02.002.
The inhibitory effects of cannabidiol on systemic malignant tumors.

Brain

Mol Cancer Ther. 2010 Jan;9(1):180-9. doi: 10.1158/1535-7163.MCT-09-0407. Epub 2010 Jan 6.
Cannabidiol enhances the inhibitory effects of delta9-tetrahydrocannabinol on human glioblastoma cell proliferation and survival.

J Pharmacol Exp Ther. 2004 Mar;308(3):838-45. Epub 2003 Nov 14.
Antitumor effects of cannabidiol, a nonpsychoactive cannabinoid, on human glioma cell lines.

Br J Pharmacol. 2005 Apr;144(8):1032-6.
Cannabidiol inhibits human glioma cell migration through a cannabinoid receptor-independent mechanism.

PLoS One. 2013 Oct 21;8(10):e76918. doi: 10.1371/journal.pone. 0076918. eCollection 2013.
Cannabidiol, a non-psychoactive cannabinoid compound, inhibits proliferation and invasion in U87-MG and T98G glioma cells through a multitarget effect.

Breast

J Pharmacol Exp Ther. 2006 Sep;318(3):1375-87. Epub 2006 May 25.
Antitumor activity of plant cannabinoids with emphasis on the effect
of cannabidiol on human breast carcinoma.

Mol Cancer Ther. 2011 Jul;10(7):1161-72. doi:
10.1158/1535-7163.MCT-10-1100. Epub 2011 May 12.
Cannabidiol induces programmed cell death in breast cancer cells by
coordinating the cross-talk between apoptosis and autophagy.

Breast Cancer Res Treat. 2011 Aug;129(1):37-47. doi: 10.1007/
s10549-010-1177-4. Epub 2010 Sep 22.
Pathways mediating the effects of cannabidiol on the reduction of
breast cancer cell proliferation, invasion, and metastasis.

Mol Cancer Ther. 2007 Nov;6(11):2921-7.
Cannabidiol as a novel inhibitor of Id-1 gene expression in aggressive
breast cancer cells.
file://localhost/message/%253CA6705605-3D1A-43FC-BDFC-
FFBCCAE851CB@whatwomenmustknow.com%253E

Colon

Phytomedicine. 2014 Apr 15;21(5):631-9. doi: 10.1016/j.phymed.
2013.11.006. Epub 2013 Dec 25.
Inhibition of colon carcinogenesis by a standardized Cannabis sativa
extract with high content of cannabidiol.

J Mol Med (Berl). 2012 Aug;90(8):925-34. doi: 10.1007/
s00109-011-0856-x. Epub 2012 Jan 10.
Chemopreventive effect of the non-psychotropic phytocannabinoid
cannabidiol on experimental colon cancer.

Leukemia

Mol Pharmacol. 2006 Sep;70(3):897-908. Epub 2006 Jun 5.
Cannabidiol-induced apoptosis in human leukemia cells: A novel role
of cannabidiol in the regulation of p22phox and Nox4 expression.

Mol Pharmacol. 2006 Sep;70(3):897-908. Epub 2006 Jun 5.
Cannabidiol-induced apoptosis in human leukemia cells: A novel role
of cannabidiol in the regulation of p22phox and Nox4 expression.
file://localhost/message/%253Ca06002000d5fa0cabf623@
%255B10.1.1.5%255D%253E

Lung

FASEB J. 2012 Apr;26(4):1535-48. doi: 10.1096/fj.11-198184. Epub
2011 Dec 23.
Cannabidiol inhibits lung cancer cell invasion and metastasis via
intercellular adhesion molecule-1.

Mol Cancer Ther. 2013 Jan;12(1):69-82. doi:
10.1158/1535-7163.MCT-12-0335. Epub 2012 Dec 7.
COX-2 and PPAR-γ confer cannabidiol-
induced apoptosis of human lung cancer cells.

Pharm Res. 2010 Oct;27(10):2162-74. doi: 10.1007/
s11095-010-0219-2. Epub 2010 Jul 29.
Decrease of plasminogen activator inhibitor-1 may contribute to the
anti-invasive action of cannabidiol on human lung cancer cells.

Prostate

Br J Pharmacol. 2013 Jan;168(1):76-8. doi: 10.1111/j.
1476-5381.2012.02121.x.
Towards the use of non-psychoactive cannabinoids for prostate
cancer.

Curr Oncol. 2016 Mar; 23(Suppl 2): S15–S22.
Published online 2016 Mar 16. doi: 10.3747/co.23.2893
PMCID: PMC4791143
In vitro and *in vivo* efficacy of non-psychoactive cannabidiol in
neuroblastoma.

Chronic Pain and Neuropathic Pain

Hemp Extract has been traditionally used for thousands of years to treat various types of pain.

Chronic pain is defined as any pain that lasts for three months or more. It can originate in the brain, nerves and muscles or at a site of trauma.

Hemp Extract stimulates the CB2 receptors to block the release of chemical messengers that are causing the inflammation and swelling at the site of injury.

When a nerve is irritated, pinched or injured, the experience is one of burning, sharp, shocking, tingling nerve pain. It is called neuropathy. These neuropathic pain messages are sent from the site of the injury up to the brain, where they are perceived as pain. This is a common condition in diabetes or with herniated disks.

Hemp Extract has been shown to be effective in managing pain in several ways. It interacts with the receptors in the immune system and brain. These receptors are tiny proteins attached to cells that receive a message to respond to chemical signals from different stimuli. When Hemp Extract interacts with these receptors, it creates a pain-relieving and anti-inflammatory effect.

Hemp Extract also works by modifying the perception of pain in the brain. A study showed that Hemp Extract proved to be tenfold more potent than morphine in a wide range of neuron-mediated pain.

Evidence suggests that cannabinoids are beneficial for nerve pain modulation by inhibiting neuronal transmission in pain pathways.

Hemp Extract will also work synergistically with opioids, reducing the need for opioid medication by 30 percent or more.

Hemp Extract can be used in a topical application to treat localized pain, inflammation and swelling. For a more systemic effect, it is recommended to take an oral Hemp Extract formula as well as a topical formula.

Curr Pain Headache Rep. 2014 Oct;18(10):451. doi: 10.1007/s11916-014-0451-2.
Cannabinoids for neuropathic pain.

Curr Med Res Opin. 2007 Jan;23(1):17-24.
Meta-analysis of cannabis based treatments for neuropathic and multiple sclerosis-related pain.

Curr Pain Headache Rep. 2014 Oct;18(10):451. doi: 10.1007/s11916-014-0451-2.
Cannabinoids for neuropathic pain.

Int J Biochem Cell Biol. 2014 Oct;55:72-8. doi: 10.1016/j.biocel.2014.08.007. Epub 2014 Aug 21.
Neuropathic orofacial pain: cannabinoids as a therapeutic avenue.

Eur J Pharmacol. 2007 Feb 5;556(1-3):75-83. Epub 2006 Nov 10.

The non-psychoactive cannabis constituent cannabidiol is an orally effective therapeutic agent in rat chronic inflammatory and neuropathic pain.

Br J Pharmacol. 2014 Feb;171(3):636-45. doi: 10.1111/bph.12439. Cannabidiol inhibits paclitaxel-induced neuropathic pain through 5-HT(1A) receptors without diminishing nervous system function or chemotherapy efficacy.

Br J Pharmacol. 2011 Feb;162(3):584-96. doi: 10.1111/j. 1476-5381.2010.01063.x.
Non-psychoactive cannabinoids modulate the descending pathway of antinociception in anaesthetized rats through several mechanisms of action.

Curr Neuropharmacol. 2006 Jul;4(3):239-57.
Role of the cannabinoid system in pain control and therapeutic implications of the management of acute and chronic pain episodes.

Neuropathic Pain

Curr Med Res Opin. 2007 Jan;23(1):17-24.
Meta-analysis of cannabis based treatments for neuropathic and multiple sclerosis-related pain.

Int J Biochem Cell Biol. 2014 Oct;55:72-8. doi: 10.1016/j.biocel. 2014.08.007. Epub 2014 Aug 21.
Neuropathic orofacial pain: cannabinoids as a therapeutic avenue.

Eur J Pharmacol. 2007 Feb 5;556(1-3):75-83. Epub 2006 Nov 10.
The non-psychoactive cannabis constituent cannabidiol is an orally effective therapeutic agent in rat chronic inflammatory and neuropathic pain.

Ther Clin Risk Manag. 2008 Feb;4(1):245-59.
Cannabinoids in the management of difficult to treat pain.

Curr Neuropharmacol. 2006 Jul;4(3):239-57.
Role of the cannabinoid system in pain control and therapeutic implications of the management of acute and chronic pain episodes.

Depression

Hemp Extract offers relief from depression without the accompanying side effects from antidepressant medications. Results are also experienced within days rather than weeks or more as is the case with antidepressants.

Hemp Extract has shown the ability to increase the availability of the neurotransmitter serotonin. Low serotonin levels contribute to depression.

Through brain scans of people with depression and anxiety, researchers found a smaller hippocampus, a part of the brain that is in charge of cognition and memory formation. Evidence from animal trials has demonstrated that Hemp Extract stimulates the hippocampus and triggers new neuron creation — called *neurogenesis*. This is another powerful method that can address depression and anxiety.

The use of Hemp Extract for depression is really an effective option for this serious mood disorder and is certainly a much safer alternative than antidepressants.

CNS Neurol Disord Drug Targets. 2014;13(6):953-60.
Antidepressant-like and anxiolytic-like effects of cannabidiol: a chemical compound of Cannabis sativa.

Curr Pharm Des. 2014;20(23):3795-811.
Endocannabinoid signaling in the etiology and treatment of major depressive illness.

Lipids Health Dis. 2012 Feb 28;11:32. doi:
10.1186/1476-511X-11-32.
Serum contents of endocannabinoids are correlated with blood
pressure in depressed women.

CNS Neurol Disord Drug Targets. 2014;13(6):953-60.
Antidepressant-like and anxiolytic-like effects of cannabidiol: a
chemical compound of Cannabis sativa.

Br J Pharmacol. 2010 Jan;159(1):122-8. doi: 10.1111/j.
1476-5381.2009.00521.x. Epub 2009 Dec 4.
Antidepressant-like effects of cannabidiol in mice: possible
involvement of 5-HT1A receptors.

Diabetes and Metabolic Syndrome

Diabetes affects 29 million Americans. This serious condition is most common among people over 65 years old, but it also affects younger people. Children as young as 10 years of age are now being diagnosed with diabetes.

Diabetes is a group of metabolic disorders that are associated with an insulin production defect that leads to the inability of the body to regulate sugar levels in the blood. With type 1 diabetes, a person is unable to produce their own insulin and is dependent on medication. People with type 2 diabetes produce insufficient insulin, and their bodies can't maintain a healthy insulin level. If either type is left untreated, it can lead to kidney failure, amputation, blindness and death. Fortunately, studies have shown that cannabidiol may help with or mitigate symptoms of diabetes.

Chronic inflammation has long been known to play a key role in the development of insulin resistance and therefore type 2 diabetes. Research has found that the anti-inflammatory properties of Hemp Extract could treat this inflammation and therefore improve metabolism.

Dr. Raphael Mechoulam found that the therapeutic effects of Hemp Extract could be tailored to different endocannabinoid receptors in the body, including those in the pancreas. The pancreas regulates blood glucose levels, releasing insulin to combat high levels of blood glucose.

Research has shown the many modes of action by which Hemp Extract can help people with diabetes, including the following:

- Stabilizing blood sugars
- Arterial anti-inflammatory properties
- Neuroprotective effects that help prevent inflammation of nerves and reduce the pain of neuropathy
- "Anti-spasmodic agents" help relieve muscle cramps and the pain of gastrointestinal (GI) disorders
- Acting as a vasodilator to help keep blood vessels open and improve circulation
- Lowering blood pressure — which is vital for diabetics
- Helping calm diabetic restless leg syndrome (RLS)

- In addition to the use of Hemp Extract, an effective program should also include a sugar-free, nutrient-rich diet along with daily exercise.

Am. J or Med July 2013 Volume 126, Issue 7, Pages 583–589
The Impact of Marijuana Use on Glucose, Insulin, and Insulin Resistance among US Adults.

Orv Hetil. 2012 Apr 1;153(13):499-504. doi: 10.1556/OH. 2012.29308.
[The potential use of cannabidiol in the therapy of metabolic syndrome].

Handb Exp Pharmacol. 2011;(203):75-104. doi: 10.1007/978-3-642-17214-4_4.
Cannabinoids and endocannabinoids in metabolic disorders with focus on diabetes.

Endocrine Disorders

The *endocrine system* refers to the collection of glands of an organism that secrete hormones directly into the circulatory system to be carried toward a distant target organ. The major endocrine glands include the pineal gland, pituitary gland, pancreas, ovaries, testes, thyroid gland, parathyroid glands, hypothalamus, gastrointestinal tract and adrenal glands.

In addition to the specialized endocrine organs, many other organs that are part of other body systems, such as bone, kidney, liver, heart and gonads, have secondary endocrine functions. For example, the kidney secretes endocrine hormones such as erythropoietin and renin.

According to studies, Hemp Extract treats disorders affecting the endocrine system. One of its major effects in the endocrine system is its ability to decrease the level of cortisol in blood plasma. The lower level of this hormone results in reduction of stress and lessening of symptoms of hormonal imbalance.

Most hormonal issues as well as chronic disease are caused or exacerbated by stress. By reducing the stress response, the endocrine system is able to regain balance and proper functioning.

Neuroimmunomodulation. 2010;17(3):153-6. doi:
10.1159/000258711. Epub 2010 Feb 4.
Endocannabinoid system participates in neuroendocrine control of homeostasis.

Endocr Rev. 2006 Feb;27(1):73-100. Epub 2005 Nov 23.
The emerging role of the endocannabinoid system in endocrine regulation and energy balance.

Endocr Relat Cancer. 2008 Jun;15(2):391-408. doi: 10.1677/
ERC-07-0258.
Endocannabinoids in endocrine and related tumours.

Pharmacol Ther. 2011 Mar;129(3):307-20. doi: 10.1016/j.pharmthera.
2010.10.006. Epub 2010 Nov 3.
Role of the endocannabinoid system in food intake, energy homeostasis and regulation of the endocrine pancreas.

J Psychopharmacol. 2012 Jan;26(1):114-24. doi:
10.1177/0269881111408458. Epub 2011 Aug 8.
The role of the endocannabinoid system in the neuroendocrine regulation of energy balance.

Endometriosis

Endometriosis is a common and often debilitating condition. This condition is characterized by the overgrowth of tissue that lines the uterus, called the *endometrium*. Side effects of endometriosis include chronic pelvic pain, painful menstrual periods, and painful intercourse, gastrointestinal upsets such as diarrhea and constipation and nausea. Some severe cases result in infertility.

There is growing evidence that endometriosis is not really so much a hormonal condition as it is an autoimmune disease. Endometriosis fulfills most of the classification criteria for autoimmune diseases, including blood markers of inflammatory cytokines and tissue-specific autoantibodies. It also frequently occurs with other autoimmune conditions such as autoimmune thyroid disease and inflammatory bowel disease.

One of the main benefits of Hemp Extract is its anti-inflammatory property, which helps to relax the abdominal muscles as well as ease painful menstrual cramps.

Pain from endometriosis can occur at any time in a woman's cycle. Since Hemp Extract acts as an analgesic, it alleviates pain throughout the body, e.g., from bowel movements, backaches, headaches, etc.

Hemp Extract also combats the nausea that sometimes accompanies intense cramping and pain. It can also provide powerful relief from anxiety and depression.

Hemp Extract has also shown the ability to slow the growth of endometrial tissue.

Endometriosis is linked to an endocannabinoid deficiency. In fact, hormone imbalances and a lack of proper endocannabinoid tone may contribute to excess inflammation associated with endometriosis.

Hemp Extract can be considered another part of a healing program for endometriosis. The combination of its anti-inflammatory and immunomodulatory effects engages with the body's immune system, improving endocannabinoid tone and reducing pain and inflammation.

Reprod Sci. 2016 Aug;23(8):1071-9. doi: 10.1177/1933719116630414. Epub 2016 Feb 17.
Elevated Systemic Levels of Endocannabinoids and Related Mediators Across the Menstrual Cycle in Women With Endometriosis.

Hum Reprod. 2017 Jan;32(1):175-184. Epub 2016 Nov 7.
The cannabinoid receptor CB1 contributes to the development of ectopic lesions in a mouse model of endometriosis.

Free Radic Biol Med. 2011 Sep 1;51(5):1054-61. doi: 10.1016/ j.freeradbiomed.2011.01.007. Epub 2011 Jan 14.
Cannabidiol as an emergent therapeutic strategy for lessening the impact of inflammation on oxidative stress.

Am J Pathol. 2010 Dec; 177(6): 2963–2970.

doi: 10.2353/ajpath.2010.100375
Antiproliferative Effects of Cannabinoid Agonists on Deep
Infiltrating Endometriosis

Epilepsy and Seizures

Epilepsy, a condition in which people have recurrent seizures, affects
three million people. While it can affect people of all ages, it is most
commonly diagnosed in children. It is a central nervous system
condition in which the nerve cell activity in the brain is disturbed.
More than half of the cases have no known cause.

Unfortunately, in more than 30 percent of the cases, even multiple
medications aren't effective in controlling the seizures. In addition,
the side effects are often so debilitating that the patient can't continue
using the medications.

Adult onset seizure disorder is usually due to head trauma.
Medications are often ineffective and also cause serious side effects.

It has now been clinically proven that the use of Hemp Extract is
remarkably effective in alleviating the symptoms of epilepsy in
infants, children and adults. It also helps to significantly reduce the
frequency and severity of seizures.

A study conducted by the American Epilepsy Society found Hemp
Extract effective in treating epilepsy in children and adults. Hemp
Extract was also able to reduce frequency and severity of seizures.

Published May 2017 in the *New England Journal of Medicine*, the research focuses on Hemp Extract as a treatment for Dravet syndrome, a complex and hard to treat form of childhood epilepsy.

Considering how difficult epilepsy is to treat, especially in infants, this is an exciting breakthrough. The use of Hemp Extract has proven to be not only safe and effective but also affordable.

Epilepsy Behav. 2013 Dec;29(3):574-7. doi: 10.1016/j.yebeh.
2013.08.037.
Report of a parent survey of cannabidiol-enriched cannabis use in pediatric treatment-resistant epilepsy.

Cochrane Database Syst Rev. 2012 Jun 13;(6):CD009270. doi:
10.1002/14651858.CD009270.pub2.
Cannabinoids for epilepsy.

Epilepsy Behav. 2014 Dec;41:277-82. doi: 10.1016/j.yebeh.
2014.08.135. Epub 2014 Oct 1.
Cannabis, cannabidiol, and epilepsy — from receptors to clinical response.

† Endocannabinoid Research Group, Institute of Biomolecular Chemistry (ICB), National Council of Research (CNR), 80078 Pozzuoli (NA) Italy
Nonpsychotropic Plant Cannabinoids, Cannabidivarin (CBDV) and Cannabidiol (CBD), Activate and Desensitize Transient Receptor Potential Vanilloid 1 (TRPV1) Channels in Vitro: Potential for the Treatment of Neuronal Hyperexcitability

J Pharmacol Exp Ther. 2010 Feb;332(2):569-77. doi: 10.1124/jpet.
109.159145. Epub 2009 Nov 11.
Cannabidiol displays antiepileptiform and antiseizure properties in vitro and in vivo.

J Epilepsy Res. 2017 Jun 30;7(1):16-20. doi: 10.14581/jer.17003.
eCollection 2017 Jun.
Could Cannabidiol be a Treatment Option for Intractable Childhood
and Adolescent Epilepsy?

Fibromyalgia

Fibromyalgia is a chronic disorder that manifests as pain in various
parts of the body, especially in the muscular and skeletal tissue. Of
the 3 million who are affected, most are women.

Dr. Ethan Russo, a neurologist and medical researcher, postulates
that fibromyalgia is due to a deficiency of the body's
endocannabinoids. Since Hemp Extract increases the level of natural
endocannabinoids in the brain and body, he showed that Hemp
Extract reduced the pain levels in people with fibromyalgia. Hemp
Extract also improved sleep and mood, two conditions associated
with fibromyalgia.

Hemp Extract can be taken either internally or topically, applied to
painful areas of the body.

Neuro Endocrinol Lett. 2008 Apr;29(2):192-200.
Clinical endocannabinoid deficiency (CECD): can this concept
explain therapeutic benefits of cannabis in migraine, fibromyalgia,
irritable bowel syndrome and other treatment-resistant conditions?

Cochrane Database Syst Rev. 2016 Jul 18;7:CD011694. doi:
10.1002/14651858.CD011694.pub2.
Cannabinoids for fibromyalgia.

Gastrointestinal Conditions: Colitis and Crohn's Disease, Celiac Disease, Inflammatory Bowel Disease (IBD), Irritable Bowel Syndrome (IBS)

Colitis and Crohn's disease, celiac disease, inflammatory bowel disease (IBD), and irritable bowel syndrome (IBS) are classified as conditions that affect the small and large intestines. All conditions except irritable bowel disease fit into the category of inflammatory conditions.

Colitis, Crohn's disease and IBS involve not just inflammation but also irregular muscle movements and issues with water absorption in the large intestines. These issues can cause serious discomfort and a variety of other symptoms.

Research demonstrates the ability of Hemp Extract to become one of the strongest anti-inflammatory compounds currently available. Since most gastrointestinal disorders are caused or worsened by chronic inflammation, Hemp Extract is able to inhibit the production of an enzyme called fatty acid amide hydrolase (FAAH). This fatty acid essentially regulates the production (or lifespan) of endocannabinoids. When the FAAH is reduced, endocannabinoid levels are increased.

Many bowel issues are believed to be caused by endocannabinoid deficiencies. Therefore Hemp Extract is an effective treatment because it increases endocannabinoid levels.

Hemp Extract also reduces the permeability of the intestinal walls. When cells become inflamed within the stomach and intestines, they allow more fluids to pass through the gut and into the body, triggering pain, irritation and a reduction in the ability to absorb nutrients. Healing gut permeability plays a major role in reversing the wide range of gastrointestinal conditions.

Phytother Res. 2013 May;27(5):633-6. doi: 10.1002/ptr.4781. Epub 2012 Jul 20.
Cannabidiol in inflammatory bowel diseases: a brief overview.

Pharmacology. 2014;93(1-2):1-3. doi: 10.1159/000356512. Epub 2013 Dec 17.
Cannabis finds its way into treatment of Crohn's disease.

PLoS One. 2011;6(12):e28159. doi: 10.1371/journal.pone.0028159. Epub 2011 Dec 6.
Cannabidiol reduces intestinal inflammation through the control of neuroimmune axis.

Br J Pharmacol. 2010 Jun;160(3):712-23. doi: 10.1111/j. 1476-5381.2010.00791.x.
The effects of Delta-tetrahydrocannabinol and cannabidiol alone and in combination on damage, inflammation and in vitro motility disturbances in rat colitis.

Pharmacology. 2012;89(3-4):149-55. doi: 10.1159/000336871. Epub 2012 Mar 12.
Topical and systemic cannabidiol improves trinitrobenzene sulfonic acid colitis in mice.

Pharmacol Ther. 2010 Apr;126(1):21-38. doi: 10.1016/j.pharmthera. 2009.12.005. Epub 2010 Feb 1.
Cannabinoids and the gut: new developments and emerging concepts.

Eur Rev Med Pharmacol Sci. 2008 Aug;12 Suppl 1:81-93.
Cannabinoids and gastrointestinal motility: animal
and human studies.

Inflamm Bowel Dis. 2017 Feb;23(2):192-199. doi: 10.1097/MIB.
0000000000001004.
Manipulation of the Endocannabinoid System in Colitis: A
Comprehensive Review.

Eur Rev Med Pharmacol Sci. 2008 Aug;12 Suppl 1:81-93.
Cannabinoids and gastrointestinal motility: animal and human
studies.

Glaucoma

Glaucoma is a common eye condition affecting more than three million Americans. It causes optical nerve damage and, when left untreated, it can lead to blindness.

Evidence increasingly suggests that glaucoma is considered to be a neurodegenerative condition. It has a connection to other neurodegenerative diseases such as Alzheimer's disease. Studies have shown that one out of four Alzheimer's patients also has glaucoma. In fact, glaucoma appears to be a significant predictor of Alzheimer's.

Since intraocular pressure (IOP) influences the onset and progression of glaucoma, ophthalmologists prescribe treatments that target intraocular pressure. In fact, the only way to prevent vision loss (or eventual blindness) is to lower IOP levels. Depending on the severity and progression, glaucoma is treated with medications such as prescription eye drops or surgery.

Going back to the 1970s, studies have shown that cannabinoids can alleviate glaucoma-related symptoms because they lower the intraocular pressure (IOP) and have neuroprotective actions.

Hemp Extract is a promising and safe option to help people with glaucoma.

Am J Pathol. 2003 Nov;163(5):1997-2008.
Neuroprotective effect of (-)Delta9-tetrahydrocannabinol and cannabidiol in N-methyl-D-aspartate-induced retinal neurotoxicity: involvement of peroxynitrite.

J Glaucoma. 2006 Oct;15(5):349-53.
Effect of sublingual application of cannabinoids on intraocular pressure: a pilot study.

Heart Disease

Increasing evidence suggests that Hemp Extract may help with cardiovascular conditions such as heart disease and atherosclerosis.

Currently, heart disease is among the major causes of death. Heart disease is caused by blood vessels hardening and plaque buildup over time, which reduces cardiovascular function.

Plaque poses serious problems when dislodged from the vessels it is attached to. Eventually, it can travel to smaller blood vessels, where it causes blockage. Tissue function is lost in areas with decreased blood flow.

Studies have shown that Hemp Extract helps in relaxing the arterial walls. This lessens tension within the blood vessels. This, in turn, protects arteries against inflammation.

Using Hemp Extract has been proven effective as a way of reducing metabolic issues of increased glucose responses, a major factor in heart disease.

Heart disease is always associated with inflammation. The anti-inflammatory and immune-modulating abilities of Hemp Extract, as well as its antioxidant protection, reduces damage to heart tissue.

Additionally, Hemp Extract provides protection to the heart against cardiomyopathy, a condition that causes thickening and hardening of the heart muscle as well as eventual limitation of blood flow.

Hemp extract has shown to stop the production of endotoxins, pro-inflammatory cytokines that are associated with the progression of heart disease.

Arterial plaque is another significant factor in heart disease. Hemp Extract has been proven effective in decreasing plaque adhesion on the arterial walls.

To sum it up, Hemp Extract addresses the key issues contributing to heart disease: relaxing arterial walls, calming inflammation, increasing antioxidant protection, modulating immune response, and decreasing plaque buildup.

BSCR 2011 Autumn meeting abstracts
17 Cannabidiol as an anti-arrhythmic, the role of the CB1 receptors.

Br J Clin Pharmacol. 2013 Feb;75(2):313-22. doi: 10.1111/j.
1365-2125.2012.04351.x.
Is the cardiovascular system a therapeutic target for cannabidiol?

Br J Pharmacol. 2010 Jul;160(5):1234-42. doi: 10.1111/j.
1476-5381.2010.00755.x.
Acute administration of cannabidiol in vivo suppresses ischaemia-induced cardiac arrhythmias and reduces infarct size when given at reperfusion.

J Am Coll Cardiol. 2010 Dec 14;56(25):2115-25. doi: 10.1016/j.jacc.
2010.07.033.
Cannabidiol attenuates cardiac dysfunction, oxidative stress, fibrosis, and inflammatory and cell death signaling pathways in diabetic cardiomyopathy.

Am J Physiol Heart Circ Physiol. 2007 Dec;293(6):H3602-7. Epub 2007 Sep 21.
Cannabidiol, a non-psychoactive Cannabis constituent, protects against myocardial ischemic reperfusion injury.

Mol Med. 2015 Jan 6;21:38-45. doi: 10.2119/molmed.2014.00261.
Cannabidiol Protects against Doxorubicin-Induced Cardiomyopathy by Modulating Mitochondrial Function and Biogenesis.

Inflammatory Conditions

Research shows Hemp Extract can stop inflammation by activating CB2 receptors found in the endocannabinoid system.

Chronic inflammation plays a role in autoimmune diseases like arthritis, lupus, colitis and multiple sclerosis. It is also associated with pain. The inflammatory process can be a major internal process that contributes and exacerbates chronic diseases such as cancer, diabetes, heart disease, Alzheimer's, and many more.

The CB2 receptors in the hemp plant inhibit inflammation. Hemp Extract activates the CB2 receptor.

Hemp Extract contains a wide variety of substances that can help not only in stopping inflammation but also in preventing or treating ailments like liver cirrhosis, osteoarthritis or arteriosclerosis.

Hemp Extract also offers an alternative for people who have chronic pain and rely on more dangerous, habit-forming medications like opioids.

The good news is that Hemp Extract addresses many of the underlying issues that result in systemic inflammation as well chronic pain in the body.

Free Radic Biol Med. 2011 Sep 1;51(5):1054-61. doi: 10.1016/j.freeradbiomed.2011.01.007. Epub 2011 Jan 14.

Cannabidiol as an emergent therapeutic strategy for lessening the impact of inflammation on oxidative stress.
Curr Opin Clin Nutr Metab Care. 2014 Mar;17(2):130-8. doi: 10.1097/MCO.0000000000000027.
The endocannabinoid system: an emerging key player in inflammation.

Pancreas. 2013 Jan;42(1):123-9. doi: 10.1097/MPA. 0b013e318259f6f0.

Anti-inflammatory role of cannabidiol and O-1602 in cerulein-induced acute pancreatitis in mice.

AAPS J. 2009 Mar;11(1):109-19. doi: 10.1208/s12248-009-9084-5. Epub 2009 Feb 6.
Cannabinoids, endocannabinoids, and related analogs in inflammation.

Eur J Pharmacol. 2012 Mar 5;678(1-3):78-85. doi: 10.1016/j.ejphar. 2011.12.043. Epub 2012 Jan 12.
Cannabidiol, a non-psychotropic plant-derived cannabinoid, decreases inflammation in a murine model of acute lung injury: role for the adenosine A(2A) receptor.

PLoS One. 2011;6(12):e28159. doi: 10.1371/journal.pone.0028159. Epub 2011 Dec 6.
Cannabidiol reduces intestinal inflammation through the control of neuroimmune axis.

World J Diabetes. 2010 Mar 15;1(1):12-8. doi: 10.4239/wjd.v1.i1.12.
Diabetic retinopathy: Role of inflammation and potential therapies for anti-inflammation.

Kidney Disease

In chronic kidney disease, also known as chronic renal failure, there is a progressive loss of kidney function. Chronic kidney disease often goes undetected until the disease is in advanced stages. Almost 14 percent of people are diagnosed with chronic kidney disease.

Hemp Extract can work in many ways to help in the treatment of kidney disease:

- Blocks the inflammatory cytokines, which can adversely affect the kidneys. It also reduces the activity in the pathway responsible for the expression of genes that aid in inflammation.
- Cleanses the digestive tract.
- In a study conducted in 2002, patients showed a marked reduction in pain by the use of Hemp Extract.
- Reduces the effects of nephrotoxicity, thus improving renal function.
- Reduces headaches associated with kidney disease.

It is proven that Hemp Extract can help alleviate the symptoms of kidney disease and also help to address the underlying conditions that can result in chronic renal failure.

J Pharmacol Exp Ther. 2009 Mar;328(3):708-14. doi: 10.1124/jpet. 108.147181. Epub 2008 Dec 12.
Cannabidiol attenuates cisplatin-induced nephrotoxicity by decreasing oxidative/nitrosative stress, inflammation, and cell death.

Lymphedema

Lymphedema is a serious condition wherein large quantities of lymphatic fluid accumulate in different areas of the body. It can happen in the face, neck, groin, legs, or even the chest. It is usually caused by some kind of trauma to the body.

The main causes of this issue later in life include radiation treatments or cancer surgery, especially breast cancer. Anything that can cause a disruption to the normal flow of lymph fluids can lead to lymphedema.

It is very likely that some of the causes contributing to lymphedema include inflammation, oxidative stress and infections. It would certainly be safe to use Hemp Extract to help address some of the underlying issues. Hemp Extract has also been shown to slow down the progression of lymphedema.

Menopause

Reduction in endocannabinoid signaling may be responsible for some of the uncomfortable symptoms associated with menopause such as hot flashes, night sweats, depression, anxiety, headaches and weight gain.

Estrogen levels are linked to endocannabinoid levels, and both peak during ovulation. This does not occur during perimenopause and menopause.

An enzyme that controls estrogen levels, called fatty acid amide hydrolase (FAAH), breaks down an endocannabinoid molecule that is regulated by estrogen. In fact, activation of estrogen receptors and cannabinoid receptors found on the same cells often synergize to produce greater effects.

All parts of the endocannabinoid system are present in the human ovary, including the endocannabinoid called anandamide and its receptors, CB1 and CB2. Anandamide has a role in egg maturity and release during the menstrual cycle.

Endocannabinoid deficiency, a state in which levels of anandamide are too low, may initiate early menopause. Interestingly, underweight women or women with anorexia, who enter menopause early, also have low endocannabinoid levels. Boosting endocannabinoid levels or stimulating cannabinoid receptors with Hemp Extract may help prevent early menopause.

Anxiety and depression are often intensified during menopause. Estrogen recruits the ECS to regulate emotional response through its actions on the brain. Lowered levels of estrogen during and after menopause mean less activation of the ECS, and poor ability to respond to stress and elevate mood accordingly.

The ECS regulates the bone loss seen after menopause. Cannabinoid receptor type 2 (CB2) is found on bone cells, called *osteoblasts*. A common mutation in the gene that codes CB2 in humans, resulting in fewer CB2 receptors, is associated with osteoporosis after menopause. Supplementing with Hemp Extract helps to support healthy bone growth and repair.

Estrogen recruits the ECS to regulate emotional response and relieves anxiety and depression through its actions on the brain. The reduced estrogen levels during and after menopause cause decreased activation of the ECS, and a poor ability to respond to stress and elevate mood accordingly. Again, adding Hemp Extract as part of a daily program will assist in managing menopausal stress and moods.

Hemp Extract provides protection from breast cancer. It has been shown to kill breast cancer cells independent of its activity on cannabinoid receptors while being protective to breast cells.

It makes sense to include Hemp Extract in a program to help maintain and balance the hormonal system as well as overall hormonal health. It is also a great support to alleviate menopausal and postmenopausal symptoms.

It is well established that Hemp Extract assists with a gentle menopause experience by improving moods, reducing stress, building bones, balancing hormones, protecting brain cells, relieving headaches and migraines, and balancing the endocrine system.

Metabolic Syndrome, Weight Gain and Obesity

Metabolic syndrome is a health condition that raises your risk for diabetes, heart disease, stroke, and other health problems. It causes weight gain, particularly around the waistline, increases triglyceride levels, and raises blood pressure. These are all risk factors for chronic illness that include diabetes, strokes and cardiovascular disease.

Researchers studied the effects of Hemp Extract on immature fat cells to explore potential benefits for the treatment and prevention of obesity. They found that Hemp Extract helps reduce metabolic syndrome by:

- Stimulating genes and proteins that enhance the breakdown and oxidation of fat.
- Increasing the number and activity of mitochondria (which increases the body's ability to burn calories).
- Decreasing the expression of proteins making fat cells.

Hemp Extract induces "fat browning" i.e., converting what is normally white-colored fat tissue that stores energy into beige-colored fat tissue that burns it much more efficiently.

A study published in the *American Journal of Medicine* found that Hemp Extract was effective in lowering fasting insulin levels. It also reduced levels of insulin resistance and increased levels of HDL-C.

In addition, Hemp Extract signals the brain receptors in the ECS to modulate fat accumulation and energy intake in the body. In fact, Hemp Extract can help those who are overweight to lose excess pounds while helping those who are underweight to gain weight.

There is yet another impact that Hemp Extract has on weight. Receptors in the gastrointestinal tract, as well as in the hypothalamus, have shown a direct relationship in the reduction of hunger signals. Using Hemp Extract helps to regulate these signals.

Cannabinol and cannabidiol exert opposing effects on rat feeding patterns.
Diabetologia. 2008 Aug;51(8):1356-67. doi: 10.1007/ s00125-008-1048-2. Epub 2008 Jun 18.
The endocannabinoid system in obesity and type 2 diabetes

Cardiology. 2009;114(3):212-25. doi: 10.1159/000230691. Epub 2009 Jul 29.
Role of the endocannabinoid system in abdominal obesity and the implications for cardiovascular risk.

Handb Exp Pharmacol. 2011;(203):75-104. doi: 10.1007/978-3-642-17214-4_4.
Cannabinoids and endocannabinoids in metabolic disorders with focus on diabetes.

Migraines

A migraine is a type of vascular headache of varying intensity and is often accompanied by nausea, vomiting and sensitivity to light and sound. More than 3 million people suffer with migraines.

There are many theories as to what triggers a migraine, including hormonal changes in women, stress, caffeinated or alcoholic drinks, food additives, sensory stimuli and food sensitivities.

One compelling theory suggests that the major cause is dysregulation in the ECS. Scientists have observed several ECS mechanisms that may have an implication in migraine attacks.

Perhaps the clearest indication of endocannabinoid dysfunction contributing to migraines is a 2007 study at the University of Perugia and published in the *Journal of Neuropsychopharmacology*. Researchers measured endocannabinoid levels in the cerebrospinal fluid of patients with chronic migraines, finding significantly lower amounts of the cannabinoid anandamide, concluding that this "may reflect an impairment of the endocannabinoid system in these patients, which may contribute to chronic head pain."

Research has proven that Hemp Extract brings balance to the ECS. Dr. Ethan Russ, a pioneering scientist in the endocannabinoid field, has postulated that "cannabidiol is an endocannabinoid modulator; in other words, when given chronically it actually increases the gain of the system.... So, if there's too much activity in a system, homeostasis requires that it be brought back down. If there's too little, it's got to come up. And that's what cannabidiol can do as a promoter of endocannabinoid tone."

Thus, increasing the body's level of natural cannabinoids by using Hemp Extract can reduce or even resolve the occurrence of migraines. In addition, Hemp Extract may also reduce the severity of a migraine attack.

You can apply a topical Hemp Extract to the area of the head and neck that is experiencing pain as well as using an oral Hemp Extract to increase endocannabinoid tone.

Neuro Endocrinol Lett. 2008 Apr;29(2):192-200.
Clinical endocannabinoid deficiency (CECD): can this concept explain therapeutic benefits of cannabis in migraine, fibromyalgia, irritable bowel syndrome and other treatment-resistant conditions?

J Headache Pain. 2011 Apr;12(2):177-83. doi: 10.1007/ s10194-010-0274-4. Epub 2011 Feb 18.
Effects of anandamide in migraine: data from an animal model.

Headache. 2013 Mar;53(3):447-58. doi: 10.1111/head.12025. Epub 2012 Dec 20.
Cannabinoids and hallucinogens for headache.

Exp Neurol. 2010 Jul;224(1):85-91. doi: 10.1016/j.expneurol. 2010.03.029. Epub 2010 Mar 29.
The endocannabinoid system and migraine.

Motion Sickness and Nausea

Scientists have established that Hemp Extract has anti-nausea properties. In addition to calming feelings of nausea, it can also help with motion sickness.

Vomiting and nausea are also common symptoms among people who are undergoing chemotherapy or after surgery as well as people with viral illnesses. Evidence shows that Hemp Extract is effective in relieving vomiting and nausea cause by these treatments.

Motion sickness and stress are also associated with impaired endocannabinoid activity. Hemp Extract has shown the ability to enhance signaling in the ECS. In addition, Hemp Extract was proven to work faster to relieve motion sickness than most conventional drugs.

PLoS One. 2010 May 21;5(5):e10752. doi: 10.1371/journal.pone.0010752.
Motion sickness, stress and the endocannabinoid system.

Eur J Pharmacol. 2014 Mar 15;727:99-105. doi: 10.1016/j.ejphar.2014.01.047. Epub 2014 Feb 4.
Dexamethasone alleviates motion sickness in rats in part by enhancing the endocannabinoid system.

Basic Clin Pharmacol Toxicol. 2008 Aug;103(2):150-6. doi: 10.1111/j.1742-7843.2008.00253.x.
The effects of cannabidiol and tetrahydrocannabinol on motion-induced emesis in Suncus murinus.

Eur J Pharmacol. 2014 Jan 5;722:134-46. doi: 10.1016/j.ejphar.2013.09.068. Epub 2013 Nov 1.

Regulation of nausea and vomiting by cannabinoids and the endocannabinoid system.

Br J Pharmacol. 2012 Apr;165(8):2620-34. doi: 10.1111/j. 1476-5381.2011.01621.x.
Cannabidiol, a non-psychotropic component of cannabis, attenuates vomiting and nausea-like behaviour via indirect agonism of 5-HT(1A) somatodendritic autoreceptors in the dorsal raphe nucleus.

Psychopharmacology (Berl). 2011 Jun;215(3):505-12. doi: 10.1007/s00213-010-2157-4. Epub 2011 Jan 18.
Interaction between non-psychotropic cannabinoids in marihuana: effect of cannabigerol (CBG) on the anti-nausea or anti-emetic effects of cannabidiol (CBD) in rats and shrews.

Br J Pharmacol. 2011 Aug;163(7):1411-22. doi: 10.1111/j. 1476-5381.2010.01176.x.
Regulation of nausea and vomiting by cannabinoids.

Multiple Sclerosis

Multiple sclerosis (MS) is an autoimmune disorder that attacks the myelin sheath covering nerves.

Symptoms vary in severity based on the amount and location of nerve damage. Symptoms include tremor, lack of coordination, unsteady gait, tingling or pain in body parts, numbness or weakness in one or more limbs, partial or complete loss of vision in one or both eyes, double vision or blurred vision, slurred speech, fatigue, dizziness and heat sensitivity.

Hemp Extract impacts MS via several mechanisms. It decreases the autoimmune inflammatory destruction of the myelin sheath. Hemp

Extract modulates the immune response, halting the assault on the central nervous system. This helps to slow or even stop the progression of MS and decreases the associated symptoms of pain and muscle stiffness.

Hemp Extract also improves serotonin levels in the brain, improving sleep and depressed mood, both common issues with MS patients.

Oral Hemp Extract can be used daily along with topical Hemp Extract, which is applied to tight or painful muscle areas.

Neurobiol Dis. 2013 Nov;59:141-50. doi: 10.1016/j.nbd.2013.06.016. Epub 2013 Jul 11.
Cannabidiol provides long-lasting protection against the deleterious effects of inflammation in a viral model of multiple sclerosis: a role for A2A receptor.

Curr Med Res Opin. 2007 Jan;23(1):17-24.
Meta-analysis of cannabis based treatments for neuropathic and multiple sclerosis-related pain.

Fitoterapia. 2017 Jan;116:77-84. doi: 10.1016/j.fitote.2016.11.010. Epub 2016 Nov 25.
Target regulation of PI3K/Akt/mTOR pathway by cannabidiol in treatment of experimental multiple sclerosis.

Eur Neurol. 2016;76(5-6):216-226. Epub 2016 Oct 13.
Tetrahydrocannabinol:Cannabidiol Oromucosal Spray for Multiple Sclerosis-Related Resistant Spasticity in Daily Practice. CNS Neurol Disord Drug Targets. 2017;16(5):541-553. doi: 10.2174/1871527316666170413114210.
Neurological Aspects of Medical Use of Cannabidiol.

Neurogenesis – Creating New Brain Cells

Neurogenesis is the process by which the brain renews and upgrades itself. It is through neurogenesis that new brain cells are created. These neurons process and carry information to appropriate destinations throughout the body. It was once theorized that it is impossible to grow new brain cells. However, this theory has been overturned and it is now known that it is indeed possible to regenerate brain cells at any age.

A study originally published in the *International Journal of Neuropharmacology* points to Hemp Extract as a cause of neurogenesis. Specifically, this birth of new neurons occurred in the hippocampus, an area typically associated with conscious memory and navigation. The neurogenesis research suggests that Hemp Extract helps to regulate stress levels. Hemp Extract is typically known for relieving pain, stress, anxiety and a number of other conditions.

The most recent of these benefits was found by a group of researchers from Brazil and Spain. They aimed to determine the effect neurogenesis has on Hemp Extract's anxiety relief. They first caused mice to be stressed. Two hours later, each day, they gave the mice 30 mg of Hemp Extract and recorded their levels of neurogenesis. Their findings were that Hemp Extract spurred an increase in neuron production and battled the effects of chronic, unpredictable stress.

Birthing new brain cells is of immense importance for living a healthy and vital life, at any age. This is another reason to use Hemp Extract on a regular basis.

Curr Neuropharmacol. 2013 May; 11(3): 263–275.
Published online 2013 May. doi: 10.2174/1570159X11311030003
PMCID: PMC3648779
Cannabinoids, Neurogenesis and Antidepressant Drugs: Is there a Link?

Br J Pharmacol. 2015 Aug; 172(16): 3950–3963.
Published online 2015 Jun 16. doi: 10.1111/bph.13186
PMCID: PMC4543605
The role of cannabinoids in adult neurogenesis.

Neurodegenerative Disease and Conditions

A neurodegenerative disease is characterized by progressive degeneration and/or death of nerve cells. It affects the neurons in the human brain, which are building blocks of the nervous system.

Alzheimer's, Parkinson's and Huntington's are all neurodegenerative diseases. Severe head traumas or repeated concussions can also cause neurodegenerative conditions.

Recent research indicates that Hemp Extract plays a role in helping to reduce or prevent further decline in neurodegenerative conditions and improve cognitive function.

Hemp Extract stimulates the CB2 receptors found on immune system cells in the brain. This results in a decreased inflammatory response. Therefore, Hemp Extract has the potential to decrease the extent of damage caused by inflammatory response.

Hemp Extract can also improve the symptoms of tremor, spasm, depression, anxiety and pain that can accompany many of these conditions.

Findings suggest that Hemp Extract is therapeutically beneficial for traumatic brain injuries, spinal cord injuries, spinal cord diseases and strokes.

Hemp Extract's neuroprotective properties are also potentially beneficial in helping prevent and limit the progression of neurological disorders, such as amyotrophic lateral sclerosis (ALS), epilepsy, multiple sclerosis (MS), and Parkinson's disease.

Neurotherapeutics. 2015 Oct;12(4):699-730. doi: 10.1007/s13311-015-0377-3.
Molecular Targets of Cannabidiol in Neurological Disorders.

CNS Neurosci Ther. 2009 Winter;15(1):65-75. doi: 10.1111/j.1755-5949.2008.00065.x.
Cannabidiol: a promising drug for neurodegenerative disorders?

Br J Clin Pharmacol. 2013 Feb;75(2):323-33. doi: 10.1111/j.1365-2125.2012.04341.x.
Cannabidiol for neurodegenerative disorders: important new clinical applications for this phytocannabinoid?

Psychopharmacology (Berl). 2012 Feb;219(4):1133-40. doi: 10.1007/s00213-011-2449-3. Epub 2011 Aug 26.
Memory-rescuing effects of cannabidiol in an animal model of cognitive impairment relevant to neurodegenerative disorders.

Pharmacol Res. 2016 Oct;112:119-127. doi: 10.1016/j.phrs.
2016.01.033. Epub 2016 Feb 1.
Cannabidiol, neuroprotection and neuropsychiatric disorders.

Prog Neuropsychopharmacol Biol Psychiatry. 2017 Apr 3;75:94-105.
doi: 10.1016/j.pnpbp.2016.11.005. Epub 2016 Nov 23.
Cannabidiol reduces neuroinflammation and promotes
neuroplasticity and functional recovery after brain ischemia.

 J Cell Biochem. 2017 Jun;118(6):1531-1546. doi: 10.1002/jcb.25815.
Epub 2016 Dec 29.
Cannabidiol Activates Neuronal Precursor Genes in Human Gingival
Mesenchymal Stromal Cells.

Neuropharmacology. 2017 Apr;116:151-159. doi: 10.1016/
j.neuropharm.2016.12.017. Epub 2016 Dec 21.
Cannabidiol reduces brain damage and improves functional recovery
in a neonatal rat model of arterial ischemic stroke.

CNS Neurol Disord Drug Targets. 2017;16(5):541-553. doi:
10.2174/1871527316666170413114210.
Neurological Aspects of Medical Use of Cannabidiol.

Parkinson's Disease

Parkinson's disease is classed as a neurodegenerative disease of the central nervous system, affecting 6 million people worldwide, most of whom are over 60.

One of the key roles of the ECS is to regulate the lifespan of a cell, especially in the central nervous system. In neurodegenerative diseases, the ECS has a neuroprotective effect and helps to mitigate the neuronal damage occurring in Parkinson's.

While current Parkinson's medication seeks to redress the depletion of dopamine, the main focus of current cannabinoid research is into the neuroprotective, antioxidant and anti-inflammatory properties of Hemp Extract.

Hemp Extract scavenges the free radicals that are associated with Parkinson's.

Hemp Extract improves cell survival and the expression of proteins related to growth of neuronal cell parts. It prevents toxin-induced decline of nerve growth factor, which may help in neuron regeneration.

Hemp Extract is also effective in reducing inappropriate muscle tension, which is another symptom of Parkinson's disease.

Since Parkinson's disease is difficult to treat, Hemp Extract shows great promise as part of a more comprehensive protocol.

J Psychopharmacol. 2014 Nov;28(11):1088-98. doi:
10.1177/0269881114550355. Epub 2014 Sep 18.
Effects of cannabidiol in the treatment of patients with Parkinson's disease: an exploratory double-blind trial.

Br J Pharmacol. 2011 Aug;163(7):1365-78. doi: 10.1111/j.
1476-5381.2011.01365.x.
Prospects for cannabinoid therapies in basal ganglia disorders.

Brain Res. 2007 Feb 23;1134(1):162-70. Epub 2006 Dec 28.
Evaluation of the neuroprotective effect of cannabinoids in a rat model of Parkinson's disease: importance of antioxidant and cannabinoid receptor-independent properties.

Front Neurosci. 2016 Aug 2;10:321. doi: 10.3389/fnins.2016.00321. eCollection 2016.
Cannabinoid Type 2 (CB2) Receptors Activation Protects Against Oxidative Stress and Neuroinflammation Associated Dopaminergic Neurodegeneration in Rotenone Model of Parkinson's Disease.

CNS Neurol Disord Drug Targets. 2017;16(5):541-553. doi: 10.2174/1871527316666170413114210.
Neurological Aspects of Medical Use of Cannabidiol.

Premenstrual Syndrome (PMS)

Premenstrual syndrome (PMS) is a disorder that affects many women during the one to two weeks before menstruation.

Symptoms can include abdominal bloating, acne, anxiety, backache, breast swelling and tenderness, cramps, depression, food cravings, fatigue, headaches, insomnia, joint pain, nervousness, skin eruptions, water retention and personality changes. It is estimated that 70 percent of women experience some variation of PMS symptoms.

Hemp Extract's well-researched ability to help with both pain management and mood stabilization make it an ideal option for those looking for a solution that can help alleviate many PMS symptoms. Additionally, Hemp Extract's calming properties help to improve sleep, by reducing the effects of stress and anxiety on the body.

Ther Clin Risk Manag. 2008 Feb; 4(1): 245–259.
Published online 2008 Feb.
PMCID: PMC2503660
Cannabinoids in the management of difficult to treat pain.

Neurosci Biobehav Rev. 2014 May;42:116-31. doi: 10.1016/ j.neubiorev.2014.02.006. Epub 2014 Feb 26.
A critical role for prefrontocortical endocannabinoid signaling in the regulation of stress and emotional behavior.

Behav Neurosci. 2008 Dec;122(6):1378-82. doi: 10.1037/a0013278.
The nonpsychoactive cannabis constituent cannabidiol is a wake-inducing agent.

Post-Traumatic Stress Disorder (PTSD)

Post traumatic stress disorder (PTSD) affects more than 2 million Americans. It develops in response to a shocking, frightening, or dangerous event. Although our active-duty military and veterans represent the lion's share of PTSD cases, PTSD also affects police officers, firefighters, EMS personnel, victims of dangerous crimes such as rape, and people who have been involved in accidents and catastrophic natural disasters.

Hemp Extract is an effective PTSD treatment, delivering acute and long-lasting effects in reducing fear memories.

PTSD and anxiety are triggered by "adverse memories." We store memories of a traumatic or emotional event in the part of our brain called the hippocampus. For most people, these adverse memories will eventually fade away. However, rather than dissipating, memories caused by traumatic events will recur in dreams as well as becoming activated by stimulating events. This results in the release of major stress hormones, creating anxiety, insomnia, nightmares, flashbacks, depression, nervousness, etc.

Studies have proven that Hemp Extract is able to decrease the responsiveness of the hippocampus to stored adverse memories. When these traumatic memories are inactivated, the body can return to a more balanced and properly regulated system.

Hemp Extract can help to reduce or alleviate the effects of PTSD in the following ways:

- Blocks mood receptors
- Regulates pain receptors
- Promotes better sleep
- Helps to enhance extinction learning
- Regulates stress hormones

Considering that most traditional treatments for PTSD are ineffective, Hemp Extract offers great promise as a safe and effective way to help heal PTSD.

Psychoneuroendocrinology. 2013 Dec;38(12):2952-61. doi: 10.1016/j.psyneuen.2013.08.004. Epub 2013 Sep 10.
Reductions in circulating endocannabinoid levels in individuals with post-traumatic stress disorder following exposure to the World Trade Center attacks.

Neuropsychopharmacology. 2005 Mar;30(3):516-24.
Enhancing cannabinoid neurotransmission augments the extinction of conditioned fear.

Neuropsychopharmacology. 2014 Jul;39(8):1852-60. doi: 10.1038/npp.2014.32. Epub 2014 Feb 12.
Modulation of fear memory by dietary polyunsaturated fatty acids via cannabinoid receptors.

J Psychiatr Res. 2012 Nov;46(11):1501-10. doi: 10.1016/j.jpsychires.2012.08.012. Epub 2012 Sep 11.
Cannabidiol blocks long-lasting behavioral consequences of predator threat stress: possible involvement of 5HT1A receptor.

Curr Pharm Des. 2014;20(13):2212-7.
Cannabinoid modulation of fear extinction brain circuits: a novel target to advance anxiety treatment Mol Neurobiol. 2007 Aug;36(1): 92-101. Epub 2007 Aug 17.
The endocannabinoid system and extinction learning.

Neuropharmacology. 2013 Jan;64:389-95. doi: 10.1016/j.neuropharm.2012.05.039. Epub 2012 Jun 9.
A current overview of cannabinoids and glucocorticoids in facilitating extinction of aversive memories: potential extinction enhancers.

Perm J. 2016 Fall;20(4):108-111. doi: 10.7812/TPP/16-005. Epub 2016 Oct 12.
Effectiveness of Cannabidiol Oil for Pediatric Anxiety and Insomnia as Part of Posttraumatic Stress Disorder: A Case Report.

Schizophrenia and Psychosis

Affecting more than 200,000 Americans every year, schizophrenia is a severe long-term disorder that adversely affects how a person thinks, feels and behaves. It is believed that the disorder is related to an imbalance in the neurotransmitter-involving chemical reactions that occur in the brain.

Hemp Extract has anti-psychotic effects. A recent study found Hemp Extract might be able to treat some of the symptoms of schizophrenia that are seemingly resistant to existing medications. In addition, Hemp Extract does not alter body weight or food intake, which are common side effects of antipsychotic drug treatment.

Braz J Med Biol Res. 2006 Apr;39(4):421-9. Epub 2006 Apr 3.
Cannabidiol, a Cannabis sativa constituent, as an antipsychotic drug.

Eur Neuropsychopharmacol. 2014 Jan;24(1):51-64. doi: 10.1016/ j.euroneuro.2013.11.002. Epub 2013 Nov 15.
Cannabidiol as a potential treatment for psychosis.

Transl Psychiatry. 2012 Mar 20;2:e94. doi: 10.1038/tp.2012.15.
Cannabidiol enhances anandamide signaling and alleviates psychotic symptoms of schizophrenia.

Curr Pharm Des. 2012;18(32):5131-40.
A critical review of the antipsychotic effects of cannabidiol: 30 years of a translational.

Curr Pharm Des. 2014;20(13):2194-204.
Cannabinoids and schizophrenia: therapeutic prospects.

Neurosci Biobehav Rev. 2017 Apr;75:157-165. doi: 10.1016/ j.neubiorev.2017.02.006. Epub 2017 Feb 7.
Neuronal and molecular effects of cannabidiol on the mesolimbic dopamine system: Implications for novel schizophrenia treatments.

Sleep Disorders

Insomnia is a major heath problem. In the United States, some 70 million people suffer from insomnia, insufficient sleep or other sleep disorders.

Hemp Extract has the ability to reduce anxiety, which can be helpful in reducing sleep difficulties and improving sleep quality. Hemp Extract increases overall sleep time and improves insomnia. It has also has been shown to reduce insomnia in people who suffer from chronic pain.

Hemp Extract not only makes falling asleep easier, it also influences the sleep cycle. Sleep is divided into multiple cycles with different phases. Hemp Extract increases the third phase, which is the phase of deep sleep.

In addition, Hemp Extract decreases the duration of REM sleep, which is a phase of light sleep in which dreaming occurs. By reducing REM sleep, people dream less, memory is improved, and symptoms of depression are decreased.

In smaller doses, Hemp Extract can stimulate alertness and reduce daytime sleepiness, which is important for daytime performance and for the strength and consistency of the sleep-wake cycle.

Hemp Extract may help reduce REM behavior disorder in people with Parkinson's disease. REM behavior disorder is a condition that causes people to act out physically during dreaming and REM sleep.

Typically, during REM, the body is largely paralyzed. In REM behavior disorder, this paralysis doesn't occur, leaving people free to move — which can lead to disruptive sleep and to possibly injuring themselves or their sleeping partners.

Growing scientific literature alerts us to the many health consequences from lack of deep, restful sleep. Lack of sleep also impairs the ability to function optimally on a daily basis. A safe solution such as Hemp Extract offers relief for a sleep-deprived society.

PLoS One. 2014 Feb 10;9(2):e88672. doi: 10.1371/journal.pone.
0088672. eCollection 2014.
Endocannabinoid modulation of cortical up-states and NREM sleep.

PLoS One. 2016 Mar 31;11(3):e0152473. doi: 10.1371/journal.pone.
0152473. eCollection 2016.
Endocannabinoid Signaling Regulates Sleep Stability.

Current Psychiatry ReportsApril 2017, 19:23|
Cannabis, Cannabinoids, and Sleep: a Review of the Literature.

Stress

Of all the systems regulated by the ECS, its role in regulating stress is one of the most important.

Endocannabinoid signaling is found throughout the key areas related to stress, in particular the Hypothalamic-Pituitary-Adrenal (HPA) Axis, which is responsible for controlling cortisol and other stress hormones.

Endocannabinoid receptors have also been discovered in the amygdala, part of the limbic system crucially involved in emotions and memory, in particular fear.

A functioning ECS in the HPA axis and amygdala allows the body to cope with high stress levels. When there is an endocannabinoid deficiency, there is an inability to adapt to chronic stress.

As a stress reducer, Hemp Extract works by reducing the body's defensive responses to stressful events such as raised heart rate, blood pressure, and anxiety.

Proc Natl Acad Sci U S A. 2010 May 18;107(20):9406-11. doi: 10.1073/pnas.0914661107. Epub 2010 May 3.
Endogenous cannabinoid signaling is essential for stress adaptation.

Neurosci Biobehav Rev. 2008 Aug;32(6):1152-60. doi: 10.1016/j.neubiorev.2008.03.004. Epub 2008 Mar 18.
Regulation of endocannabinoid signaling by stress: implications for stress-related affective disorders.

J Neurosci. 2010 Nov 10;30(45):14980-6. doi: 10.1523/JNEUROSCI.4283-10.2010.
Functional interactions between stress and the endocannabinoid system: from synaptic signaling to behavioral output.

J Exp Biol. 2014 Jan 1;217(Pt 1):102-8. doi: 10.1242/jeb.089730.
Neuromodulators, stress and plasticity: a role for endocannabinoid signalling.

Semin Immunol. 2014 Oct;26(5):380-8. doi: 10.1016/j.smim.2014.04.001. Epub 2014 May 29.
Stress regulates endocannabinoid-CB1 receptor signaling.

Neuropsychopharmacology. 2014 Mar;39(4):919-33. doi: 10.1038/npp.2013.292. Epub 2013 Oct 21.
Cannabinoid receptor activation prevents the effects of chronic mild stress on emotional learning and LTP in a rat model of depression.

Neuropsychopharmacology. 2013 Jul;38(8):1521-34. doi: 10.1038/npp.2013.51. Epub 2013 Feb 20.
Cannabinoids ameliorate impairments induced by chronic stress to synaptic plasticity and short-term memory.

Strokes and TIAs

The American Heart Association notes that by 2030, almost 4 percent of adults will experience a stroke.

Hemp Extract is proving to play a major role in the prevention of and recovery from strokes.

Cerebral ischemia, or inadequate blood supply to the brain, caused by a stroke or heart failure can cause severe damage. Blood circulation is usually restored as quickly as possible in the emergency room, but secondary ischemia/reperfusion injury is common. Inflammation often occurs, causing oxidative-stress-induced damage in the areas deprived of blood, oxygen, and nutrients.

Hemp Extract can help alleviate the symptoms of stroke, whether it is a transient ischemic attack or hemorrhagic and ischemic stroke.

Transient ischemic stroke, or TIA, is a temporary decrease in the blood supply of the brain. This may occur in people who have diabetes or hypertension. The brain cells recover after the temporary decrease in blood supply.

Hemp Extract has neuroprotective properties, which helps to prevent brain cell death. Also, it has anti-inflammatory properties that prevent autoimmune-like attacks to tissues and blood vessels in the brain. In addition, Hemp Extract has antioxidant compounds, which help clear the blood and the blood vessels of dead cells and toxins.

One other important feature of Hemp Extract is its ability to lower blood cholesterol by increasing protective high-density lipoproteins (HDL).

Am J Physiol Heart Circ Physiol. 2007 Dec;293(6):H3602-7. Epub 2007 Sep 21.
Cannabidiol, a non-psychoactive Cannabis constituent, protects against myocardial ischemic reperfusion injury.

Neuroreport. 2004 Oct 25;15(15):2381-5.
Cannabidiol prevents infarction via the non-CB1 cannabinoid receptor mechanism.

Stroke. 2005 May;36(5):1077-82. Epub 2005 Apr 21.
Cannabidiol prevents cerebral infarction via a serotonergic 5-hydroxytryptamine1A receptor-dependent mechanism.

Neuropharmacology. 2017 Apr;116:151-159. doi: 10.1016/j.neuropharm.2016.12.017. Epub 2016 Dec 21.
Cannabidiol reduces brain damage and improves functional recovery in a neonatal rat model of arterial ischemic stroke.

MEDICAL BENEFITS OF HEMP EXTRACT
Hemp Health Revolution

Legal in every

100%

State in the US.

Supported by over

23,000

Studies World-Wide

40%

Hemp extract
constitutes up to
40% of the plant.

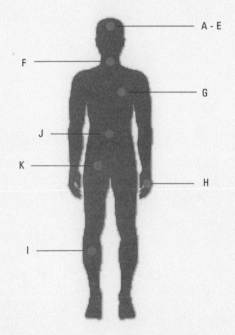

A - E

F

G

J

K

H

I

0%

Hemp extract has NO
psycho-euphoric effects

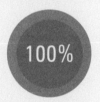

100%

100% all-natural

A	Relieves Anxiety and Depression	G	Reduces Risk of Artery Blockage
B	Reduces Stress	H	Reverses Cell Damage
C	Neuroprotective	I	Relieves Aches and Pain
D	Promotes Brain Growth	J	Improves Gut Health
E	Increases Memory	K	Improves Bone Density
F	Balances Hormones		

These are only a few of the medical benefits hemp extract has to offer. Author Sherrill Sellman goes into great detail about the incredible things hemp extract can do for your mental *and* physical health in her book, *Hemp Health Revolution*.

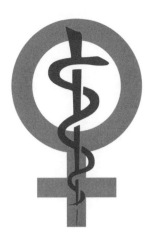

"A woman's health is her capital."

-Harriet Beecher Stowe

CHAPTER 6: HEMP EXTRACT AND WOMEN'S HEALTH

There's no doubt about it. Women face many more challenges, when it comes to their hormonal and overall health, than men do. In fact, women are four times more likely to have migraines, anxiety, irritable bowel disease and fibromyalgia.

There is a new understanding of why women are more vulnerable. It all has to do with our ECS and the fact that women are three times more vulnerable to an endocannabinoid deficiency than men.

Hemp Extract is proving to be a panacea for the many health challenges that so many women experience. The following are some of the ways that Hemp Extract can help to support women to address many of their health issues as well as to regain their health.

1. Eases Premenstrual Symptoms

Hemp Extract is able to lessen or alleviate all the major PMS symptoms including reducing inflammation that contributes to headaches/migraines, menstrual cramps, upset stomachs, and physical sensitivities. Hemp Extract naturally elevates mood, balancing mood swings and reducing depression and anxiety. It also enhances deep sleep.

2. Enhances Fertility

The ECS plays a crucial role in regulating a broad range of physiological processes, including reproductive fertility.

3. Eases Perimenopausal and Menopausal Symptoms

The ECS regulates the endocrine system. Symptoms associated with perimenopause and menopause is related to an endocannabinoid deficiency. Estrogen levels are linked to endocannabinoid levels. Since the ECS also regulates body temperature, it helps with hot flashes and night sweats. It also supports other symptoms associated with perimenopause and menopause, such as mood shifts, sleep issues, pain, cognitive impairment and low energy.

Hemp Extract can help to balance hormone levels, including estrogen, by restoring proper ECS tone.

The ECS also helps to regulate bone loss seen after menopause. The CB2 cannabinoid receptor is found in bone cells, and when there are fewer coded CB2 receptors after menopause, it leads to osteoporosis.

4. Helps Prevent Osteoporosis and Builds Bone

Hemp Extract activates the cannabinoid receptor that balances the bone remodeling process. It can help prevent bone loss. The ECS heals fractures and promotes the development of new bone tissues.

5. Helps to Prevent Breast Cancer and Reduce Treatment Symptoms

Research has shown that Hemp Extract effectively kills breast-cancer cells while sparing healthy cells. Studies show that Hemp Extract may support apoptosis (programmed cell death) by ridding the body of old and damaged cells.

Hemp Extract has been proven to minimize the side effects of chemotherapy and radiation. It increases appetite, decreases nausea, and promotes restful sleep, all of which support healing.

6. Reduces Autoimmune Diseases

Women comprise 75 percent of patients diagnosed with an autoimmune disorder. Fortunately, new research suggests that Hemp Extract may be an effective treatment for the symptoms of autoimmune disorders. It also helps to calm an overactive immune system, limiting the production of the pro-inflammatory molecules.

7. Provides Relief for Anxiety and Depression

Women are twice as likely as men to suffer from anxiety disorders. One recent study showed that Hemp Extract lessened anxiety and distress when taken just before an anxiety-provoking public speaking performance. While Hemp Extract has been proven to combat social anxiety disorder, it can also help to quickly alleviate general anxiety symptoms.

Hemp Extract has now also been found to be able to successfully and effectively treat depression.

8. Helps with Chronic Pelvic Pain

Hemp Extract reduces chronic pain by lowering inflammation. Conditions such as endometriosis are also considered to be an autoimmune condition, which are helped with Hemp Extract.

J Pharmacol Exp Ther. 2006 Sep;318(3):1375-87. Epub 2006 May
Antitumor activity of plant cannabinoids with emphasis on the effect of cannabidiol on human breast carcinoma.

Mol Cancer Ther. 2011 Jul;10(7):1161-72. doi:
10.1158/1535-7163.MCT-10-1100. Epub 2011 May 12.
Cannabidiol induces programmed cell death in breast cancer cells by coordinating the cross-talk between apoptosis and autophagy.

Mol Cancer Ther. 2007 Nov;6(11):2921-7.
Cannabidiol as a novel inhibitor of Id-1 gene expression in aggressive breast cancer cells.

Curr Neuropharmacol. 2010 Sep;8(3):243-53. doi:
10.2174/157015910792246173.
Cannabinoid receptors as target for treatment of osteoporosis: a tale of two therapies.

Acta Psychiatr Scand. 2011 Oct;124(4):250-61. doi: 10.1111/j.
1600-0447.2011.01687.x. Epub 2011 Mar 9.
Endocannabinoid system dysfunction in mood and related disorders.

Hum Fertil (Camb). 2007 Dec;10(4):207-16.
Regulation of female fertility by the endocannabinoid system.

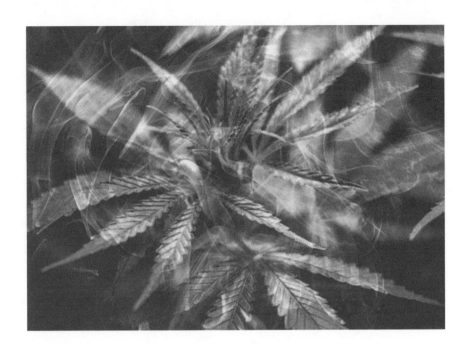

"Hemp Extract is the perfect way to raise our ECS tone naturally."

- Dr. Gregory L. Smith, MD, MPH

Author, *CBD: What You Need to Know*

CHAPTER 7: HEMP EXTRACT — HELPING TO SOLVE THE OPIOID EPIDEMIC

The United States is in the throes of an opioid epidemic, as more than 3 million Americans have become dependent on or abused prescription pain pills and street opioid drugs. Opioids are drugs formulated to replicate the pain-reducing properties of opium. They include both legal painkillers such as morphine, oxycodone or hydrocodone prescribed by doctors for acute or chronic pain, as well as illegal drugs such as heroin or illicitly made fentanyl, which is 100 times more powerful than morphine.

The Department of Health and Human Services has declared the opioid crisis a public health emergency. According to the American Academy of Pain Management, more than 100 million Americans suffer from chronic pain.

Drug overdose deaths have exceeded 59,000, the largest annual jump ever recorded in the United States.

A report recently released by the White House stated, "The opioid epidemic we are facing is unparalleled. The average American would likely be shocked to know that drug overdoses now kill more people than gun homicides and car crashes combined."

The search continues to seek solutions to the most pressing problems: providing effective, non-addictive options for pain as well as helping to manage withdrawal and recovery for the long term.

Hemp Extract is proving to have a major role to play in the opioid epidemic. It's not just the well-documented effects of Hemp Extract for pain, but Hemp Extract also has the ability to act directly on the opioid receptors.

Hemp Extract has shown to be highly effective in relieving the symptoms of addiction. Opioids produce a sense of euphoria, acting on the brain's reward pathways. After a period of time, they desensitize these pathways, which require more to achieve the same effect. Sudden withdrawal leads to intense symptoms such as pain, nausea, vomiting and anxiety.

Hemp Extract is a solution for helping people to manage withdrawal symptoms. Most people tend to think of opioid addiction as occurring at the level of opioid receptors in the brain. However, multiple neurological systems are involved – systems with which Hemp Extract also interacts.

A study investigated Hemp Extract's effects on drug cravings in heroin-dependent individuals. Basically, they gave heroin addicts a dose of Hemp Extract or placebo on three consecutive days. They then showed them opioid-related or neutral video cues and measured cue-induced drug craving. Hemp Extract decreased cravings and anxiety at all time points.

In other words, it was demonstrated that Hemp Extract was able to diminish cravings and anxiety triggered by drug-associated cues. This is key, because drug relapse in recovering addicts often follows exposure to such cues.

In addition, it was believed that Hemp Extract might have a "long-term impact on synaptic plasticity." This essentially means that the addicted brain had undergone a kind of rewiring that could reduce cravings and relapse on a more long-term basis.

It's exciting to learn that Hemp Extract not only has the ability to reduce inflammation associated with chronic pain but also is a safe and non-addictive solution to ease the symptoms of withdrawal as well as reducing the cravings associated with the use of an addictive substance.

At this time of an opioid emergency, Hemp Extract certainly needs to be acknowledged as part of the solution.

Planta Med. 2017 Aug 9. doi: 10.1055/s-0043-117838. [Epub ahead of print] Effects of Cannabidiol on Morphine Conditioned Place Preference in Mice.

JAMA Intern Med. 2014 Oct;174(10):1668-73. doi: 10.1001/jamainternmed.2014.4005.
Medical cannabis laws and opioid analgesic overdose mortality in the United States, 1999-2010.

Neurotherapeutics
October 2015, Volume 12, Issue 4, pp 807–815 | Cite as
Early Phase in the Development of Cannabidiol as a Treatment for Addiction: Opioid Relapse Takes Initial Center Stage.

Safety and pharmacokinetics of oral cannabidiol when administered concomitantly with intravenous fentanyl in humans.

Volume 40, Issue 3, p124–127, March 2017
Cannabidiol: Swinging the Marijuana Pendulum From 'Weed' to Medication to Treat the Opioid Epidemic
Leafly.com/news/science-tech/high-cbd-cannabis-pain-and-opioid-addiction

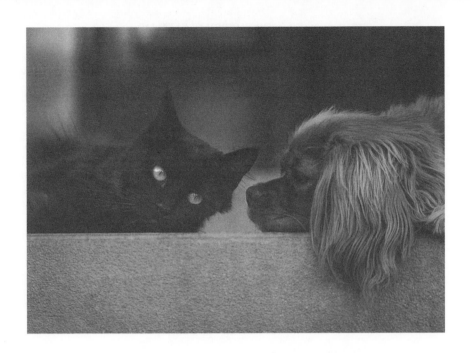

"Until one has loved an animal a part of
one's soul remains unawakened."

- Anatole France

CHAPTER 8: HEMP EXTRACT FOR PETS

Since our furry friends also have an endocannabinoid system, Hemp Extract can provide great relief for their many health challenges, as it does for their human companions. Dogs, cats, rabbits, horses and other livestock can safely be given Hemp Extract to support their health. Even hamsters, birds, ferrets and snakes have been known to benefit.

Instead of relying on pharmaceutical medications, with their long list of side effects (just like in humans), the use of Hemp Extract offers an effective, affordable and safe option.

Hemp Extract has demonstrated to be successful for a wide variety of animal issues:

- Reduces nausea and vomiting
- Calms anxiety, agitation and nervousness
- Improves appetite
- Reduces inflammation and chronic pain
- Eliminates allergies
- Cancer
- Reduces convulsions, seizures and muscle spasms
- Promotes a healthy digestive tract
- Promotes comfort at the end of life
- Improves neurological function

In fact, just about any benefit that Hemp Extract offers humans will also be effective for animals.

Calming Anxious Animals

Our pets are easily affected by stress and anxiety. It may be due to previous abuse or trauma. Perhaps they have separation or abandonment anxiety when left alone. Or, it could just be the animal's nature. Whatever the cause, Hemp Extract can come to the rescue.

Anxiety and stress often result from loud noises such as a thunderclap or fireworks. It can send dogs and cats into such distress that they are terrified for hours.

Hemp Extract would be a natural solution for this reaction. When an anxiety-inducing situation is about to occur, such as a thunderstorm, give your pet a dose of Hemp Extract. This will help them to relax and show decreased signs of nervousness and agitation.

The use of Hemp Extract as a treatment for dog anxiety has produced some amazing results. Hemp Extract has produced almost miraculous changes with some pets. Anecdotes abound of dogs that have suffered from so much chronic anxiety that they have never integrated properly into their human family, yet they experienced dramatic turnarounds when treated with Hemp Extract.

Settling Nausea

Hemp Extract can be a huge help in overcoming nausea, vomiting or a sensitive stomach.

For instance, cats that are having a hard time adjusting to a new food or who have a weak stomach can benefit from some Hemp Extract.

Since cats can be notoriously fickle with their food and may avoid it if it smells different than normal, you may want to introduce the Hemp Extract slowly over a period of time.

Helping with Pain and Arthritis

Hip and joint pain is a common challenge for older dogs. This is particularly true for breeds that are especially prone to certain painful diseases such as herniated discs, hip inflammation, arthritis, and intervertebral disc disease. It goes without saying that pain will limit a dog's mobility.

Of course, cats often deal with painful conditions too as they get older. In fact, most animals, large or small, will be vulnerable to pain with age.

Racehorses often retire with severe injuries at a young age. Chronic pain can significantly shorten a horse's lifespan by forcing them to favor one leg at the expense of others. Hemp Extract can be used both topically and orally to help reduce inflammation and accelerate healing of painful joints.

Hemp Extract is a powerful anti-inflammatory that can quickly reduce pain and improve the ability to be more active. Unlike prescribed medications, Hemp Extract is totally safe and fast-acting for reducing any kind of pain and arthritis.

Reducing Allergic Reactions

Another wonderful benefit of Hemp Extract is its ability to address the problem of an allergic reaction. Allergies may cause a variety of reactions, which also include skin issues such as dermatitis, mange and alopecia.

Just like in humans, pets experience an allergic reaction when their immune system views a substance (like pollen, chemicals or insect saliva) as a threat and increases the production of histamines in the body's systems. Animals show itching either by chewing or licking their skin or scratching. Commonly affected are the cheeks, belly, feet, the armpit region and ears.

Hemp Extract will calm an overactive immune system that contributes to allergic reactions. It will help to reduce itching and skin irritations.

A Natural Solution for Cancer

Hemp Extract has been found to have an anti-tumor effect. It has even been shown to stop cancer cells from growing and can cause increased tumor cell death.

Some more progressive veterinarians are now including Hemp Extract in their protocols for their patients. Australian vet Edward Bassingthwaighte discovered how Hemp Extract could be a critical part of his holistic veterinary practice. One of his patients was a senior Staffordshire terrier who had a 6 cm mammary tumor and metastasis that disappeared in 3 months and didn't come back.

Palliative Care for Pets

Hemp Extract can contribute to a dignified final phase of life for your pet. It will help to create a calm, peaceful emotional state while reducing pain.

Treating Seizures and Epilepsy

It's estimated that up to 5% of dogs suffer from seizures. Most dogs with seizures are put on drugs such as phenobarbital and potassium bromide. While these drugs may help control the seizures, they can be extremely harmful to the dog's liver and other organs. And the drugs don't work in all cases.

Hemp Extract has proven to be another safe and effective alternative treatment for this condition.

Keeping Your Pet Young and Healthy

Just like their human companions, pets can benefit from Hemp Extract's ability to increase endocannabinoid tone, which will support optimal health and enhance the body's ability to repair and regenerate at any age. Your pet deserves a natural anti-aging program, too!

How to Give Hemp Extract to Animals

There are many ways to administer Hemp Extract to animals. It can be added to their food, mixed in with their favorite treats, or dropped directly into their mouths.

If you have a picky pet, then introduce it slowly in smaller doses with their food or with a treat.

Hemp Extract is available as a liquid or in a capsule. There are also some pet products that come in the form of Hemp Extract treats.

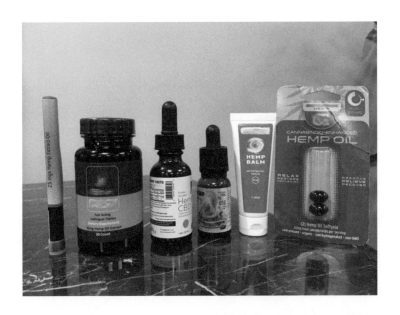

"Compared to any other oral-based method, liposomal technology delivers more of the actual nutrient to your body."

CHAPTER 9: CHOOSING THE BEST HEMP EXTRACT PRODUCT

As Hemp Extract products become more widely known and appreciated, many more formulations are entering the marketplace. While there are now a variety of choices, the question is always, "Which ones are really the best?" In sorting through the many options, it is important to know the bioavailability, the source of the hemp plant, the extraction method, the purity, the delivery system, and the potency.

What Is Bioavailability?

Bioavailability is the proportion of the active ingredients that is absorbed and utilized by the body. No matter how beneficial a medicinal substance may be, if it is not bioavailable, it is useless. The higher the bioavailability, the more effective the product will be. Bioavailability of Hemp Extract products varies greatly depending on the type of delivery system, e.g. capsule, spray, vaporized, etc. The information in this chapter will help you understand how to choose the best Hemp Extract product.

Sourcing the Hemp Plant

Until recently, the hemp plant was sourced from Europe because it was illegal to grow hemp in the United States. But due to new federal regulations, farmers in many states are now growing agricultural hemp. There are agricultural hemp farms that are dedicated to growing organic hemp.

Be sure to seek out an organically grown Hemp Extract formula.

What Is the Best Extraction Method?

The CO_2 extraction method is by far the best method. It uses carbon dioxide under high pressure and extremely low temperatures to isolate, preserve and maintain the purity of the medicinal oil. This process requires expensive equipment, but the end product is safe, potent and free of chlorophyll.

Other extraction methods either use toxic solvents or the process creates an end product that has a very unpleasant taste and is inefficiently absorbed.

When choosing a Hemp Extract product, always check to be sure the CO_2 extraction method was used.

What Is the Most Effective and Absorbable Delivery System?

There is a big difference between merely ingesting a substance such as Hemp Extract and efficiently absorbing its active ingredients.

When nutrients and beneficial plant phytochemicals enter the body, they have certain requirements before they can be readily absorbed and utilized by the cells. As much as 85 percent of the bioactive nutrients in Hemp Extract can be destroyed in the digestive process.

The usual delivery methods for Hemp Extract include capsules, tinctures and concentrates. However, Hemp Extract formulas have their own particular challenge when it comes to efficient absorption. Hemp oil, in its natural form, is a dense, sticky oil. Getting any oil-based substance to pass through a cell wall is a challenge, as the absorption rate can be greatly reduced. This means that very little of the active ingredients can be absorbed by the cells. So, you may need to take a higher dose in order to benefit, or the formula may not be absorbed at all.

Liposomal Delivery System

Enter liposomal delivery technology. Liposomes are tiny hollow spheres that have the ability to carry both water-soluble and fat-soluble compounds very efficiently through the body and into cell membranes. You can also think of them as very small, nano-sized packets that are the delivery system allowing for rapid absorption of nutrients into the cell.

A liposome is nature's own delivery system. In fact, the science of liposomes copied what nature had already created!

It all started with mother's milk! It was discovered that mother's milk contains liposomes. It is the way nature is able to ensure that the life-sustaining nutrients in mother's milk are easily absorbed by the infant. Liposomes also protect the nutrients as they pass through the stomach and are delivered into the small intestine.

Over 50 years ago, science found the way to duplicate nature's highly efficient delivery system by creating liposomal technology. Liposomes are effective because they are able to increase nutrient solubility and improve nutrient bioavailability, and they are also very stable within the body.

At present, liposomes are the most bioavailable way to deliver nutrients into the cells.

The reason liposomes are so effective is that they can be absorbed very quickly through a cell wall, either orally or topically. They enhance the effectiveness of Hemp Extract due to this super-efficient delivery method. By attaching to hemp oil molecules and transporting them to their destination, liposomes are a perfect delivery solution for achieving rapid results.

Therefore, liposomal technology allows the Hemp Extract to be absorbed 6-10 times more efficiently than the capsule or liquid oil delivery methods.

However, not all liposomes are created equal. Many liposome products on the market use toxic solvents in their processing. An inferior-quality liposome will use low grades of phospholipids, e.g. raw lecithin. Liposomes also are less effective when exposed to heat and oxygen.

The process of making stable, quality liposomes is tricky. The inherent stability of the phospholipids and nutrients also plays an important role in the overall stability of liposomal products. Getting all of these things exactly right, then ensuring that the liposomes and nutrients remain stable throughout the product's shelf life, is key.

Fortunately, there is a high-quality liposome technology called HempSorb™. It is the most advanced liposomal technology presently available for Hemp Extract formulations.

HempSorb™ liposomal technology uses high-quality phospholipids; it also does not use heat, pressure, toxic solvents or any GMO ingredients.

HempSorb™, a proprietary form of liposomes, provides the highest concentration of liposomes per dose, which makes for the most therapeutic delivery method.

What Is the Optimal Dose?

The way to dose a Hemp Extract formula should follow the old adage "start low, go slow." It is always recommended to begin with a lower dose. Your most effective dose will depend on several variables, such as your metabolism, body weight and desired effects. If you do not achieve the desired results with the initial dose within a couple of days, then increase the amount. You can do this several times over a couple of days until you find the dose that works for you.

People usually need to experiment to find the dose that is effective for them.

There is really no risk of overdose since Hemp Extract is harmless even in high concentrations and has no side effects.

If you want to improve your sleep, take Hemp Extract before bedtime. If your desired outcome is to alleviate pain or stress, it is advised to use it during the day and again in the evening before bedtime.

When dosing with Hemp Extract, the advice is to find your sweet spot — the dose that is just right to achieve your specific needs.

Ideally, Hemp Extract is best taken on an empty stomach for the most rapid absorption. However, if that is inconvenient, it can also be taken at mealtime.

Obviously, when using Hemp Extract with children, always start at a lower dose than with an adult. This is also true when using it with pets.

Always consult with your doctor before using Hemp Extract during pregnancy or while breastfeeding.

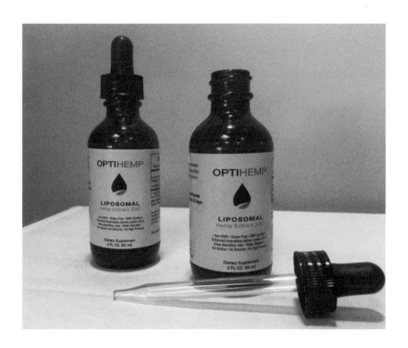

"Let the buyer beware."
Latin proverb

CHAPTER 10: FINDING YOUR WAY THROUGH THE WORLD OF HEMP EXTRACT PRODUCTS

The exciting frontier of endocannabinoid research is truly revolutionary. What's even more exciting is the further discovery that Hemp Extract, the non-psychoactive component of the hemp plant, provides such a wide spectrum of benefits — without any known side effects.

I often feel like an intrepid explorer — always in search of effective, natural solutions for the many health challenges we are facing in our 21st century world. I know answers are somewhere out there!

When I discovered the profound role the endocannabinoid system plays in every aspect of our health, I also needed to learn everything I could about the benefits of Hemp Extract.

This book is the culmination of my investigation and compilation of the published research that is propelling the great interest in Hemp Extract.

I always strive to present well-researched and documented evidence.

There is no doubt in my mind that Hemp Extract is a much-needed piece of our health puzzle.

After reading my book, I trust that you are now as excited about the healing potential of Hemp Extract formulations as I am. And you are probably ready to experience just what Hemp Extract can do for you!

But before you run out to your local health food store, there are some things I need to share with you.

As a Naturopathic Doctor, I always need to sift through all the marketing hype and false claims to find the best products for my patients. Unfortunately, the nutraceutical world is no different from any other industry. There are companies and products that are based on purity and integrity as well as companies that do not uphold these highest standards.

I certainly would not want anyone to purchase a product only to be disappointed that it did not deliver what I had promised.

So, how do you choose the best product to ensure that you get the best results?

This has been a tricky question for me because I am an objective writer and rarely make specific product recommendations.

In this case, however, I feel that I really do need to recommend a superior Hemp Extract product. And I will explain why.

The efficaciousness of a Hemp Extract formula depends on many factors, as I have explained in the previous chapter.

Just to recap: It requires sourcing organic plants, using an advanced extraction method that does not contaminate the raw material, having an effective delivery system for optimal bioavailability, and formulating a high-potency concentration of active ingredients. There is one further ingredient — an affordable price!

Based on these fundamental requirements, I am very pleased to introduce to you the OptiHemp formulas from OptiVida Health (www.OptiVidaHealth.com). Their oral liquid and topical cream formulations have met all these essential standards.

What else makes OptiHemp formulas so special?

OptiHemp formulas are made with oils extracted from non-GMO, certified organically grown hemp plants which can be traced and validated for purity from farm to finished product. They also conform to the highest industry standards for testing and purity.

In addition, OptiHemp has a clean label philosophy, which means it contains no solvents, chemicals, sugar or preservatives. It is considered a "green" Hemp Extract.

There is another important feature: OptiHemp formulas use the superior HempSorb™ liposomal delivery technology.

The best news of all is that OptiHemp formulas are very high potency. Each dose of the oral formula has 6-10 times greater bioavailability than ordinary Hemp Extract products. And it has a great-tasting, all-natural flavor.

OptiHemp submits each batch of its Hemp Extract to third-party labs for independent testing. They test for potency, any microbiological contaminations, metals, pesticides, and the unique terpene profile. The lab also tests for the existence of trace amounts of THC. To date the lab results show .00% THC — it is nonexistent in the OptiHemp extract.

The best way to take the OptiHemp liquid is to hold it in your mouth for 30-60 seconds before swallowing. This will enhance absorption directly through the mucous membranes.

Another option is to add OptiHemp to any liquid such as juice, smoothies, protein shakes, puddings, etc. Do not add to hot drinks.

The OptiHemp topical formula also contains the HempSorb™ liposomal delivery technology for deep penetration. It can be massaged into inflamed, painful joints and sore muscles.

Your pets will be happy to know that they can safely use the OptiHemp formulas for their health and wellbeing, too!

I trust that you are now ready join the Hemp Extract revolution! Everyone, of all ages, can benefit from taking Hemp Extract when needed. We truly live in an exciting time when the healing gifts from nature are so readily available to us! The ancient hemp plant has returned to help us regain our health and balance.

www.OptiVidaHealth.com.

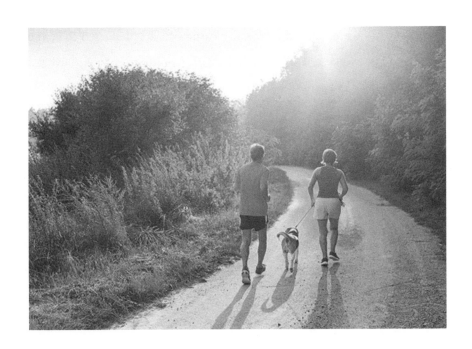

"May our words blaze the way to our future."

- *Paul Bradley Smith*

CHAPTER 11: PERSONAL TESTIMONIALS

Lifting Severe Depression

"I have dealt with periods of severe depression and overwhelming anxiety since I was a teen. I sought help from therapists, psychologists and psychiatrists. All of their methods and medications allowed me to function, but nothing allowed me to be my best self like Hemp Extract. I was introduced to a Hemp Extract tincture. I started taking it morning and night, and after a few days I noticed my

thoughts were clear, the pressure came off, and I started to remember what it was like not to be greeted with negativity each and every day."
- *Matt M.*, 33 years old

Reducing Chronic Seizures

"Seizures have plagued me since a car accident severely traumatized my brain. When they occur, I stiffen all over my body. I would often spasm uncontrollably, and I would deal with pain and confusion for hours after each event. It was suggested I try Hemp Extract. I was skeptical. On the way home I started to feel the typical precursor symptoms to my seizure. I took two droppers full of the Hemp Extract tincture and settled in for the experience. I felt my body begin to shake, but it was subtle and never got worse. I was expecting what I had felt so many times before but it just never came. I was in awe! Since then I have been using a Hemp Extract 500mg tincture as a preventative and my seizures have dropped in duration and severity. I am skeptical no more!"
- *Wendy W.*, 55 years old

Making a Huge Difference with MS Symptoms

"I am a 36-year-old woman with multiple sclerosis. I started reading about cannabidiol when I had a friend, who I often see at dialysis, mention her positive feelings regarding her Hemp Extract use. She told me that her body pain and negative sensations were relaxed. She brought me a bottle of Hemp Extract. I didn't really know where to start with it, so I just started to take it daily. I noticed some impact but I still felt pain, tingles in my feet and sensitivity to heat. I started to gradually increase the dose, and it was like the light switch flipped! My pain eased. The tingles became less frequent, and I found myself more comfortable in general! I started sleeping better, too! I am not cured, by any means, but I find things to be SO much more manageable. I attribute it to Hemp Extract."

- *Kaci T.*, 36 years old

Reducing Pain and Head Injuries for Athletes

"I have played hockey my whole life. Hockey is a tough sport, and it makes for tough players. I have used Hemp Extract for years. My brother, who lives in Colorado, turned me on to it after I hurt my knee a few years ago. After preaching to coach about this stuff, he and the coaching staff decided to make it accessible to any family who wanted to try an all-natural alternative to pain treatment. Most of us started rubbing down with Hemp Extract salve after game or in between periods. The biggest impact we saw was with concussions. The health coach would apply a Hemp Extract tincture to teammates who went down with concussions, and their symptoms seemed to fade quickly if they developed at all! Once we saw that, we knew we had something special in our bags."

- *Tyler T.*, 38 years old

Eliminating the Need for Opioids

"I was in a car accident a year ago and had a broken neck, nine broken ribs and a brain bleed. They started me on oxycodone, but after a couple of days I stopped taking it and started doing Hemp Extract and a hemp-based salve. When taking the Hemp Extract, my pain level dropped dramatically within an hour. I continue to take the Hemp Extract and the salve. It has made a huge difference, and I do not have to take opioids. I have no side effects from the hemp."

- *Mary G.*, 68 years old

Improving Depression, ADD and Memory

"I have been taking hemp oil products for over three years for depression, ADD and memory. Since taking the liposomal Hemp Extract, my brain function is much better, I have zero pain or inflammation, and my energy level is sustained all day long without feeling tired and run down. I can truly say that using Liposomal Hemp Extract has changed my life dramatically."

- *Michael S.*, 71 years old

Renewed Enjoyment for Life

"I've been on OptiHemp for about two weeks now and have a renewed enjoyment of things I used to like, such as old movies and music, plus a better sense of wellbeing. I put my dog on it, too, per your recommendation, and she is a bit more alert and perkier at times and I'm seeing a bit more of her former self."

- *Sheri*, 45 years old

Amazing Relief for Rheumatoid Arthritis

"I am in awe. My wife is not a believer that anything will help her body. She is a doubting Thomas. She was in such a flare up with her rheumatoid arthritis this morning that she couldn't open her hands. She couldn't stand straight, and her body was swollen. She was miserable. She took the Liposomal Hemp Extract, and in about 30 minutes, things slowly started to change. Her pain was gone. She still had some stiffness, but her pain was gone! She was sobbing because she could open her hands. She is astounded. She is a new person."

- *Mondo*

Severe Back Pain Resolved

"I have osteoarthritis and a herniated disk. I've been having severe back problems for well over a year. I had feared that I would get addicted to some of the strong medication that was being prescribed and wanted an alternative. I have used many methods in order to help my back issues. I've tried floating, massage, physical therapy, swimming, and stretching, to name a few. I was having continuous muscle spasms in my back. I tried the Liposomal OptiHemp liquid and thus far it's been more effective than any of the meds that the doctors have prescribed. It also helped my sleeping."

- *Barry G.,* 59 years old

PET HEALTH TESTIMONIALS

Rejuvenating a Poodle

"My three-year-old poodle, Alexia, would not eat until the Hemp Extract was added into her food. Alexia would walk up to the food bowl and smell the dog food I had placed in the bowl, but if the 500mg Hemp Extract tincture was not added, then Alexia would walk away until I added the tincture on the food. Then and only then

Alexia would run up and start eating the whole bowl of food. My precious pet now has much more energy and has a shining coat of fur, thanks to Hemp Extract."

- *Michelle*

Eliminating Hip Pain in a Great Dane

"My four-year-old Great Dane, Rex, had several hip problems and could not move around very well. He was limping and not walking well after being up for only a short while. After adding 500mg Hemp Extract tincture to Rex's food for two weeks, the results were dramatic, as Rex started to move around with a lot more vigor and flexibility. Now, after six weeks of use, Rex is walking normally, and I could not be happier with the Hemp Extract. I have been adding to his food."

- *Nick*

Extending the Life of a Cat with Cancer

"My six-year-old cat, Rocky, was diagnosed with cancer and had less than a week to live. Rocky had lost a lot of weight in the last month before I took him in to the vet to be looked at. After adding a small amount of Hemp Extract tincture to Rocky's food daily, he began to stabilize his weight and did not lose any more. Rocky was also a little more alert during his final six months of life. I miss him dearly and am glad the Hemp Extract helped him live longer than the vet thought."

- *Laura*

Calming Down an Anxious Cocker Spaniel

"My one-year-old smaller cocker spaniel mix dog, Harley, was too anxious and nervous all the time. Nothing I fed him or did would calm him down. After feeding him Hemp Extract on a daily routine, after several days Harley started to calm down and was much less anxious. After I fed Harley this daily for over a month, I consider Harley to be calm and without any anxiety, which is a big relief to me as well!"

- *Teresa*

Helping a 15-Year-Old Lab with Arthritis

"My 15-year-old lab, Zena, has been suffering from lesions and arthritis for several years. The vet told me she needed to be on medication. My friend told me about Hemp Extract and that it could help. I had no idea what Hemp Extract was, but after a week Zena was able to do things she could not do for many years, her pain level decreased, and she can go on long walks."

- *Sandy*

ABOUT THE AUTHOR

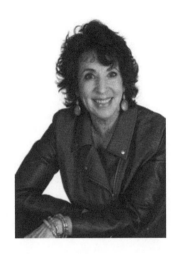

Dr. Sherrill Sellman is a doctor of traditional naturopathy and is Board Certified in Integrative Medicine. She is a psychotherapist as well, and is a leading voice in women's holistic health and wellness. Dr. Sherrill is also an internationally respected dynamic lecturer, authoritative writer and health journalist, assisting people to access truthful information and safe holistic solutions to optimize their health and wellbeing.

Dr. Sherrill is the author of three bestselling *books: Hormone Heresy: What Women MUST Know About Their Hormones, What Women MUST Know to Protect Their Daughters From Breast Cancer,* and *Chia: Return of the Ancient Seed.*

In addition, Dr. Sherrill is a much sought-after keynote speaker and educator, providing classes, seminars and workshops throughout the United States, Canada, Ireland, the UK, Australia and New Zealand. She currently maintains an international health consulting practice. Dr. Sherrill has been a guest on more than 1,400 radio and TV shows. She has written more than 500 articles for newspapers, health magazines and trade journals. For the past 15 years, Dr. Sherrill has hosted a popular weekly radio show called *What Women MUST Know,* empowering her listeners to make informed decisions regarding their health and wellbeing.

Dr. Sherrill is a passionate, inspiring and powerful voice sharing her wisdom through her books, radio show, TV appearances, blog and consultations. When not writing, consulting or lecturing, Dr. Sherrill can be found exploring interesting places and experiences around the world or bicycling through the countryside!

Visit her website at www.WhatWomenMustKnow.com

INDEX